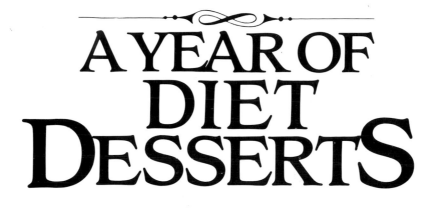

A YEAR OF
DIET
DESSERTS

A YEAR OF DIET DESSERTS

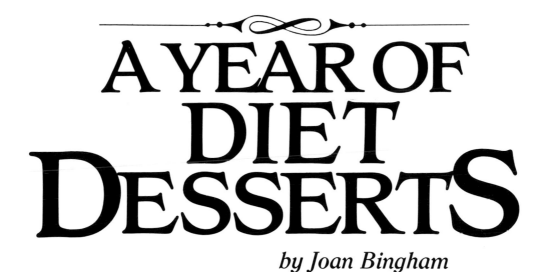

by Joan Bingham

365 Delectable Low-Calorie Treats—
A Different One for Every Day

Photography by
The Rodale Press Photography Department

Rodale Press, Emmaus, Pa.

Printed in the United States of America.

Book design: Anita G. Patterson

Illustrations: Jean Gardner

Recipes on the cover: Papaya Fluff, page 120; Saint Paddy's Day Mint Treat,
page 64; Mini Cake Rolls, page 158; Strawberry Torte, page 155.

Library of Congress Cataloging-in-Publication Data

Bingham, Joan.
    A year of diet desserts.

    Includes index.
    1. Desserts.   2. Low-calorie diet — Recipes.
I. Title.
TX773.B52   1987   641.8'6   87–12951
ISBN 0-87857-719-X

2 4 6 8 10 9 7 5 3   hardcover

Contents

Acknowledgments

Before a manuscript turns into a book, many people have to put many hours into producing it. As a free-lance author I have found that when Rodale is the publisher, all those people do a superior job.

First, I want to thank Charles Gerras, my friend and editor, whose dedication to perfection always inspires me to do my best work.

And I'm grateful to Camille Bucci, associate editor and dauntless organizer, who kept track of the seemingly thousands of details that cropped up and was instrumental in helping me resolve the problems. (And she always smiled as she did so!) A real pro!

And my heart-felt thanks to the staff of the Rodale Food Center, especially to JoAnn Brader who is not only a marvelous cook, but an absolute darling, too. She tested, suggested, and helped in so many ways. Natalie Updegrove, Beth Pianucci, Nancy Zelko, Anita Hirsch, and Diane Drabinsky also added their inestimable culinary expertise to testing the recipes, and I thank them for that.

And Anita Patterson is the one who designed this book so beautifully. Thank you, Anita.

My thanks to Marianne Laubach, Barbara Fritz, Kay Lichthardt, and Heidi Actor, the food stylists who prepared the finished dishes, dreamed up imaginative settings for them, and made sure everything looked mouth-watering and fresh.

And my thanks to Donna Hornberger, Carl Doney, Alison Miksch, Mitchell F. Mandel, Christie Tito, and Sally Ullman without whom the gorgeous, tantalizing photographs would have been impossible.

The Rodale team has done it for me a second time!

Thank you, thank you, thank you!

Introduction

Almost everyone is on a diet or watching calories, and that's no fun—especially when it means foregoing desserts, and there's a rumor among dieters that you can't eat your dessert and lose weight, too. I guess that's true if you make desserts with large amounts of the common dessert ingredients that are fattening and aren't good for you. But I think of dessert as food for the body as well as the spirit, and as with all food, I believe it should add nutrition, not just calories, to your meals. My desserts satisfy more than just your sweet tooth. I cut way down on ingredients such as egg yolks, butter, and cream that, while nutritious, are also high in fat. This means the desserts are both low calorie and wholesome. In fact, this book is proof you can enjoy a different dessert every day of the year and still stay on a diet. You probably won't want to make dessert every single day. There'll be leftovers to use, and some days you may not feel like having a sweet. But isn't it comforting to know you can have a different dessert if you want to? In a few instances, you'll notice that my servings are a bit on the small side; that is so you can enjoy a dessert that's slightly richer than most.

Nutritionally, you get out of any recipe what you put into it. I use whole grain flours for the most part, adding some unbleached white flour when it's necessary for the lightness of a cake or the flakiness of a pastry. Whole grain flours contain fewer calories than white flour. Whole wheat flour, for instance, has 400 calories per cup while a cup of all-purpose white flour contributes 455 calories to a recipe.

Handling the High-Calorie Ingredients Wisely

Sugar is a dieter's downfall: it's high in calories, and it has no nutritional benefits. Honey is the sweetener I use most often. While it's slightly higher in calories than sugar (spoon for spoon), it's also twice as sweet, so I use half the amount I would if I were sweetening with sugar. Honey isn't a very nutritious food, but it does contain small amounts of vitamins and minerals.

There are many types of honey, each with its own distinct flavor. My favorites are the readily available clover honey, wildflower honey, and orange blossom honey. I don't care for raw honey in desserts. Its strong flavor and dark color aren't compatible with delicate flavors. You'll find that desserts made with honey stay fresh and moist longer than those made with sugar.

In many of the recipes in this book, there's no sweetener added. The wonderfully natural sweetness of fruit provides all that's needed to make the dessert delicious.

Cream and even whole milk make the calories in desserts soar. I occasionally use these products in small quantities when they really are needed to achieve the results I want in a specific recipe. But as a rule, I substitute skim milk, nonfat dry milk, or plain low-fat yogurt. In most desserts the difference is barely discernible, and the calorie count and fat content are drastically reduced. These foods are excellent sources of bone-building calcium, too.

In some recipes, cream cheese takes the place of butter. With this simple substitution, you can reduce calories by 160 for every ¼ cup of cream cheese you use. And you're introducing only half as much cholesterol using cream cheese as you would with butter. In some recipes where I do use butter, the amount isn't critical. When I make sweet quick breads, for instance, I use about half of the butter a recipe ordinarily calls for, adding skim milk to obtain the proper consistency. And you can reduce the amount of shortening called for in a cake. It's surprising how little difference you'll notice in the finished product.

Yogurt, that wonderful food that's gained recognition in the past few years, can be substituted for sour cream in many desserts. This produces a dessert with substantially fewer calories. Yogurt is also a fine, low-calorie dessert topping to use in place of whipped cream. Add vanilla or almond extract and a touch of honey for flavor.

I make scrumptious cheesecakes that a dieter can eat with an easy conscience. Replacing cream cheese with the less fattening cottage cheese (or part-skim ricotta cheese) makes it possible to enjoy many variations of this popular dessert. And while these low-fat cheeses have fewer calories than their counterpart, they're still delicious, high-protein foods.

Eggs are a wonderful food. But the yolks contain the lion's share of the calories and the fat. Whenever possible, I use two egg whites in place of each whole egg called for in a recipe.

I seldom use flour as a thickener for desserts anymore, opting instead for cornstarch, tapioca, and, on occasion, eggs to provide just the desired density. And the dieter's friend, gelatin, is a frequent thickener for my recipes.

It's small wonder many people find they can't control their weight and eat desserts too. So many sweets are made with chocolate, and chocolate is over 50 percent fat and high in calories. I never use it in any form. I use carob instead. Some people don't think carob tastes like chocolate, but I maintain that when correctly used, it's difficult to tell the difference between the two. And this low-calorie chocolate taste-alike is only 2 percent fat. Its assets don't stop there. Carob contains no caffeine as chocolate does, and, because it has its own natural sweetness, you don't have to use as much sweetener in a recipe as you do with chocolate, which is quite bitter in its natural state. The secret to successful use of carob is a light touch. Its flavor is much stronger than chocolate's. I never use more than half the amount of carob I would if I were using chocolate.

Most of my cakes are so tasty in their own right, I serve them sans frostings. Others are enhanced by simple frostings or toppings, or decorated without being iced.

Sherbets, ices, and ice milks replace ice cream in the frozen desserts section of this book. I just love them! But since they're homemade and don't contain the stabilizers used in commercial ice creams, they tend to get very hard in the freezer. Removing a homemade frozen dessert from the freezer to the refrigerator an hour or two before serving time solves this problem. The time varies depending on the recipe and on the temperature of the freezer. You may have to experiment a bit.

Fruits Are a Fabulous Resource for Dieters

Most fruits are low in calories, high in fiber, rich in nutrients, and naturally, that makes them heavenly ingredients for diet desserts. Fiber has received a great deal of positive press in recent years, and it's sadly lacking in the average American diet. Fruits with edible seeds, such as figs and raspberries, are especially endowed with fiber.

Many fresh fruits are seasonal, and I try to take advantage of this by using these fruits when they're plentiful. But with modern freezing methods, frozen fruits offer a viable substitute with almost-as-good-as-fresh quality. So when I have a craving for peaches in February, I use frozen. Fresh pineapple isn't always easy to get and it doesn't work well with gelatin, so I use unsweetened canned pineapple in many of my desserts. Some fruits, such as apples, bananas, oranges, lemons, and an array of dried fruits, are in abundance year round.

This book features a fruit each month at the time that fruit is most plentiful and at its succulent best. These fruits are so delicious in their natural form that I recommend enjoying each one by itself for dessert at least once a month so you can appreciate its pure flavor.

A dessert treat I usually reserve for busy days is quickly made by folding a puree of fruit, such as peaches, into a well-beaten egg white. It's light, quick, and oh, so good. Also it's very low in calories!

Shopping Tips for the Weight-Conscious

The first rule for the weight-conscious is to be a smart shopper. Never shop when you're hungry. (You've no doubt heard that before. But it's important and so it's repeated often.) You'll be tempted by an array of foods your stomach will tell you to purchase that you know in your heart you should pass by. And always approach the market armed with a well-thought-out shopping list.

If you're buying any prepared foods, be cautious. Read the labels carefully. Ingredients are listed according to the amounts used, in descending order.

Curtail salt or sodium in any form since it causes water retention. It's abundant in prepared foods, including many where you might not expect to find it. A product marked "Low Sodium" must contain less sodium per serving than is regularly used in the same food. If the package is marked "No Salt," "No Salt Added," or "Salt Free," it has been prepared without adding any sodium. *But* that doesn't necessarily mean it's a food you should eat when you're dieting, since the food itself may have a high sodium content.

The supermarkets now boast all sorts of diet foods. Most of them contain chemicals I'd rather not use in my cooking, so I don't buy them. But it's wise to be aware of the packaging lingo. If a product is marked "Lo-Cal," it must offer no more than 40 calories per serving. And if the label reads "Calorie Reduced," the law requires that the contents be at least one-third lower in calories than the food would be normally. Of course, that still can be pretty high! The term "Sugar Free" is also misleading. While it does mean the package contains no sugar, it may contain any number of sugar substitutes. Some of them are questionable, healthwise, and others are no lower in calories than the sugar they're replacing. Even when you're shopping for honey, read the label carefully. I always select a honey that's marked "pure." If it doesn't have that word on the bottle, honey may be up to 19 percent sugar or corn syrup.

Judicious selection of dairy products to use in your desserts is a big calorie saver, indeed. The fat content is the all-important consideration here. Whole milk contains between 3.25 and 4.0 percent butterfat and at least 8.25 percent milk solids. It's a great source of protein, but it's not a diet food. "Low-fat milk" may have a range of fat from 0.5 to 2.0. Of course, the 0.5 milk is a better choice for anyone who's watching his or her weight. Low-fat milk, too, must contain at least 8.25 percent nonfat milk solids, and it still has as much protein as whole milk. But, while a glass of whole milk adds 150 calories to a recipe, a cup of skim or nonfat milk only contributes 80 calories.

Although buttermilk sounds fattening, it has only 88 calories per cup. What's sold in the markets today, however, has little resemblance to the wonderful buttermilk of years ago and I rarely use it.

Nonfat dry milk fills a variety of needs for the cook who's making low-calorie desserts. Look for "U.S. Extra Grade" on the shield. Most nonfat dry milk has been fortified with 2,000 international units of vitamin A and 400 international units of vitamin D per reconstituted quart. I always use *instant* nonfat dry milk as it dissolves much more readily than the noninstant. An added plus of nonfat dry milk is its price. It's an aid to the pocketbook as well as the waistline.

Cream is loaded with fat—light cream contains 18 to 30 percent milk fat and heavy cream has over 36 percent. I use it only very occasionally and in small quantities—to make a dessert that can't be made without it—or to adorn a dessert that's very low in calories and is much improved with just a dab of cream. I never buy ultrapasteurized cream. It does keep longer, but it also contains additives, and I find it doesn't whip properly.

Yogurt is better—dietwise—than sour cream, but it can't always be substituted for it. Yogurt has all the nutritional properties of whole milk only in *higher* amounts. I prefer to make my own yogurt, but occasionally I do buy it. Most of the yogurt in the supermarket is made from fresh, partially skimmed milk and nonfat dry milk. If the container says "low-fat yogurt," it has anywhere from 0.5 to 2.0 percent milk fat. But if it reads "nonfat yogurt," the milk fat is no more than 0.5 percent. Keep unopened yogurt stored upside down on the door of your refrigerator which is warmer than other parts of the refrigerator. Extreme cold destroys some of the good bacteria of this food.

Whether you're buying ricotta, cream cheese, or cottage cheese, check the dates on the packages in your market and select the freshest product.

I do use some butter in my dessert recipes, and I always buy the sweet, unsalted variety. When you're shopping for butter, look for the words "U.S. Grade AA" or "U.S. 93 Score."

Margarine isn't an ingredient I use, but if you prefer it, you can use it interchangeably with butter in the recipes in this book.

I'm happy to report that carob is being stocked by more and more markets. I buy both powdered carob and carob chips for use in desserts. The chips come in dark carob and milk carob flavors. The latter have a milder flavor and are my favorites. They're a little more difficult to find, but many natural foods stores stock them or will order them if you request it.

I rely heavily on spices to flavor desserts. I don't recommend buying the giant-size bottles or tins, although they may seem like a bargain, since spices lose their freshness and zing rather quickly.

Snacks

No wonder diets fail when so many of them rule out snacks. Imagine looking foward to three meager meals a day for the rest of your life! What a bleak thought. Snacks shouldn't be forbidden. In fact, they should be encouraged as an alternative to that horrible empty feeling that results in indiscriminate overeating when meal-time finally comes around. It's difficult to use restraint when you're ravenous.

There are good, acceptable snacks, and there are those that should be avoided because they're fattening. The purpose of a snack is, after all, to take the edge off your appetite. I try to keep my snacking to under 100 calories, and I prefer a sweet snack.

Once you attain your desired weight, it's easy to maintain and you don't have to starve. If you eat good nutritious foods and make meals special occasions, you'll be less apt to overeat. Don't eat on the run. Savor every mouthful, and eat sitting down at an attractively appointed table.

I find life more complete since I've found I can eat dessert as often as I like and still stay at my desirable weight. I hope you enjoy the year's recipes as much as I do.

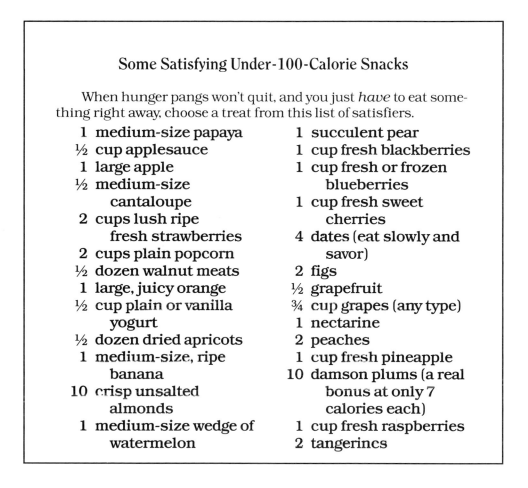

Some Satisfying Under-100-Calorie Snacks

When hunger pangs won't quit, and you just *have* to eat something right away, choose a treat from this list of satisfiers.

1 medium-size papaya	1 succulent pear
½ cup applesauce	1 cup fresh blackberries
1 large apple	1 cup fresh or frozen
½ medium-size	blueberries
cantaloupe	1 cup fresh sweet
2 cups lush ripe	cherries
fresh strawberries	4 dates (eat slowly and
2 cups plain popcorn	savor)
½ dozen walnut meats	2 figs
1 large, juicy orange	½ grapefruit
½ cup plain or vanilla	¾ cup grapes (any type)
yogurt	1 nectarine
½ dozen dried apricots	2 peaches
1 medium-size, ripe	1 cup fresh pineapple
banana	10 damson plums (a real
10 crisp unsalted	bonus at only 7
almonds	calories each)
1 medium-size wedge of	1 cup fresh raspberries
watermelon	2 tangerines

DON'T LIMIT YOUR PLEASURES!

The recipes for desserts listed on each month's calendar are contained in the chapter immediately following, although the order may change. They are arranged to provide daily variety and take advantage of seasonal fruits. But you might want to enjoy April's fancies in July or December's treats in May. Scan all the monthly calendars to become familiar with the indulgences in store throughout the year. Maybe you'd like the Saint Paddy's Day Mint Treat in February or the New Year's Day Holiday Ice Cream Bombe in August. This book was born to bring some joy into calorie control. Make the most of it!

JANUARY

Think Thin—The Mind-Body Connection to Dieting

FRUIT OF THE MONTH: **APPLES**

DESSERT OF THE MONTH: **APPLE RAISIN PIE**

DRINK OF THE MONTH: **APPLE-GRAPE DRINK**

				New Year's Day **1** HOLIDAY ICE CREAM BOMBE	**2** PEANUT PEAR PIE	**3** BLUEBERRY COBBLER
4 CHEESE COOKIES	**5** MAPLE PEAR TORTE	**6** TANGY BANANA FLUFF	**7** LIGHT LEMON GELATIN	**8** APPLE-FILLED GERMAN PANCAKES	**9** BLUEBERRY RICE PUDDING	**10** COFFEE GRANITA WITH CREAM
11 ONE SHINY RED APPLE	**12** PEACHY SCALLOP	**13** MOCK DOUGHNUT HOLES	**14** FRUITED ORANGE CUPS	Martin Luther King's Birthday **15** DREAM PIE	**16** APPLE PEAR BAKE	**17** MIXED FRUIT WITH RASPBERRY RUM SAUCE
18 APPLE AND SPICE CAKE	**19** JELLY SHAKES	**20** BANANA COCONUT ICE MILK	**21** PEACH NUT BAVARIAN	**22** STRAWBERRY FRENCH TOAST	**23** GRAPEFRUIT ORANGE PIE	**24** COCONUT THUMB PRINTS
25 PEARS À LA CRÈME	**26** BEAUTIFUL BAKED ALASKA	**27** PEARS WITH RASPBERRY SAUCE	**28** DELECTABLE CAROB CAKE	**29** APPLE RAISIN PIE ★	**30** LITE SURPRISE PUDDING	**31** EASY BAKED PEAR RINGS

Blueberry Cobbler (page 5)

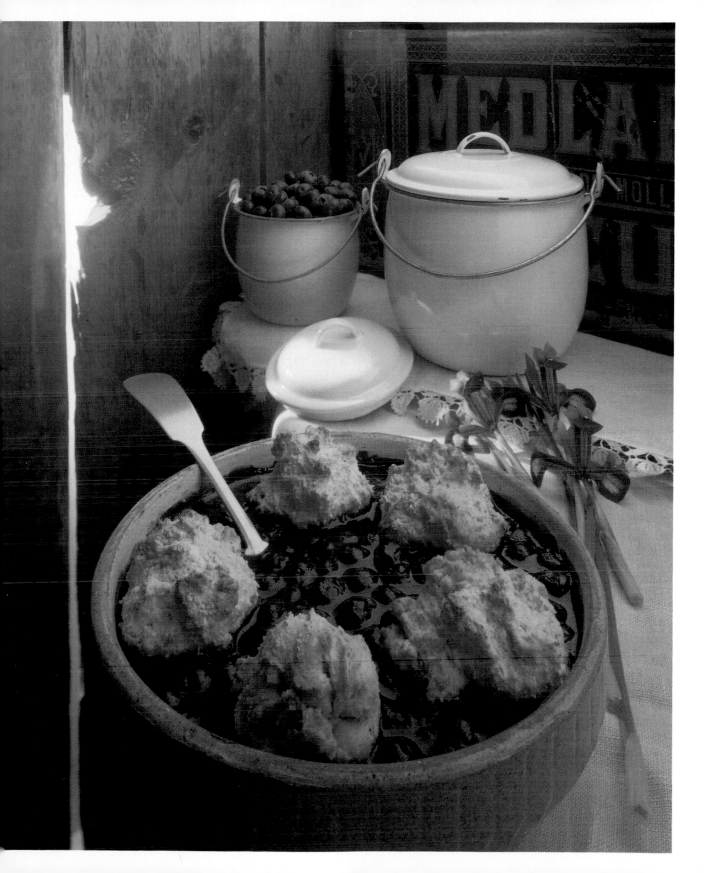

$\mathcal{I}$t's January! What a wonderful time to start a diet. There's a brand new year ahead and you're full of resolve to be better, look better, and feel better. You intend to let bad eating habits die and replace them with healthy ones. And, of course, that means shedding those extra pounds. More diets probably begin on January first than any other day of the year. But by February first most have been abandoned. One major reason for this is the negative approach so many dieters take. They expect to fail; they see themselves as failures.

Wonderful You

You're going to be successful, so the first thing you need is a good self-image. You are you. You may be overweight, but that doesn't mean you're a bad person. We all know people who are perpetually starting diets that will never last or succeed. They try every new fad diet that comes along. One month their refrigerators overflow with grapefruit, another month it's cottage cheese and pineapple. These people may lose weight for awhile, but they *always* put it back on. Most of them hate themselves for being fat. They think of themselves as losers — not of weight, but at life. They have a poor self-image.

Dr. Barbara Sternberg, a psychological consultant for Weight Watchers, says that many people actually dislike themselves so much for being overweight that they think they don't deserve to be thin. When they diet, they program themselves to fail. In order to lose weight and keep it off, you have to will yourself to succeed. You may never be a size five, but you can attain and maintain your ideal weight. That is, you can if you think you can — and then take the steps necessary to do it. But don't take on a diet that promises you will become a feather-weight overnight. That's exactly the type of diet that leads to failure. You're an okay person right now. And as you lose weight gradually, eating the right foods, along with exercise, you're going to feel better and better about yourself.

Program your subconscious to help you. If you're wishy washy about your diet and reinforce it only with thoughts of "I'll try to diet," or

"I know I should diet," your subconscious receives a weak signal. Instead say to yourself, "I will be successful at changing my eating habits to include only those foods that are good for me and will help me to attain my perfect weight." Then change your eating habits — permanently!

Does this mean you can never again enjoy all those wonderful foods you look forward to? No, it does not! I think diets in which all tempting foods are absolutely forbidden are bound to fail. There's nothing as enticing as something you are ordered to avoid forever. Most dishes that are classically made with fattening ingredients can be made in a lighter, better-for-you version. This book offers many examples of that — recipes for desserts that taste wonderful but substitute ingredients such as evaporated skim milk instead of cream, egg whites instead of whole eggs, and yogurt instead of sour cream.

Of course, substitution doesn't apply just to desserts. Light versions of most of the things you crave can be worked into your new eating program. The few dishes that just can't be made without high-calorie ingredients can be enjoyed occasionally, too. But first ask yourself, "Is this a food I really love and don't want to give up?" If you feel you can't forego it, don't abandon your diet; simply eat half as much of the treat as you would ordinarily. Eat slowly. Savor every bite. Remember this is special. As long as you don't consider any foods *absolutely* off limits, you should be able to stick to your weight loss plan.

Don't be too hard on yourself if you put on a few pounds from time to time. Be objective. You want to lose weight, your clothes are getting tight and unattractive. Proceed with a reasonable plan to remedy the situation.

In your new way of eating, it's very important to avoid letting yourself get really hungry. (No one can stick to a diet for long if it means feeling starved all the time.) And, of course, your diet must be well balanced so you'll be eating for health as well as slenderness. All of the basic food groups must be represented.

One common trait among people who have trouble losing weight is that they continue to eat when they've actually had enough, and the additional food makes them feel bloated and uncomfortable. It's essential to listen to the inner voice that says, "You've had enough." Adding bulk to your diet is a good way to make yourself feel full faster, and because fiber doesn't stay in your system as long as other substances and isn't readily absorbed, you'll get the fullness without the added weight.

Remember, dieting seldom goes smoothly. Most people have setbacks. If you binge, don't feel defeated and give up. You're entitled to stray now and then. So what, if for one meal, or one day, or even one week you reverted to your old eating habits. Forgive yourself, and go back to good, nutritional, nonfattening meals. You can regain the ground you've lost and lose the weight you've gained.

The Mental Advantages of Exercise

Exercise is important to weight loss. It not only firms your muscles and burns calories, it helps you attain self-confidence by giving you control over your body. You'll be reluctant to surrender this new sense of self, and weight control will be easier.

Auto Suggestion

Auto suggestion is a helpful tool for dieters. There are many ways you can utilize it. For instance, you can cut out a picture of a slender model—one who has a similar bone structure to yours. Paste a photograph of your face on the face in the picture and put it on the refrigerator door. Every time you go to the refrigerator, look at the picture and see yourself thin.

Another way to use auto suggestion is to buy stylish jeans, or a bathing suit in the size you aspire to. Hang it in a visible place and every time you look at it tell yourself, "It fits me perfectly."

Something for Nothing

The reward system is my favorite! Every time I put on a few extra pounds, I promise myself a special present for taking them off. The reward is never food, of course. But I might get a pair of earrings that I've been admiring, a pretty dress in my new size, or tickets to a show I've been wanting to see.

A new hobby is a great help to many dieters because it's distracting. Select something you really want to do—something you can get lost in. I found when I first took up crocheting, I would actually forget to eat.

The simple message I want to impart is: everything starts with a thought, so guard against the kind of thinking that can lead you to eating when you're not hungry. Include nonfattening foods in your diet. You can make real headway toward reaching your desired weight by adopting these two basic measures. And you don't even have to give up desserts—just use the ones in this book.

Blueberry Cobbler

3 cups unsweetened frozen blueberries, thawed
¼ cup honey
1 tablespoon cornstarch
¼ cup water
½ cup whole wheat pastry flour
½ cup unbleached white flour
1½ teaspoons baking powder
2 tablespoons butter
½ cup skim milk

Preheat oven to 375°F.

In a medium-size saucepan, combine blueberries and honey. Dissolve
cornstarch in water and add to blueberries. Cook over medium heat, stirring
constantly, until mixture thickens.

In a medium-size bowl, whisk together whole wheat pastry flour, unbleached white flour, and baking
powder. Cut butter into pieces. Add to
flour mixture and cut in with pastry
blender or 2 knives. Stir in skim milk.

Turn blueberries into a 1½-quart
casserole. Drop batter in 8 equal spoon-
fuls on top of blueberries. Bake on middle shelf of oven until batter is lightly
browned, 25 to 30 minutes.

Makes 8 servings
(160 calories per serving)

Cheese Cookies

*While these cookies aren't sweet, my
family loves them for dessert served
with a piece of fresh fruit.*

⅓ cup butter, softened
⅓ cup grated cheddar cheese
1 egg, beaten
2 tablespoons skim milk
¾ cup whole wheat pastry flour
¼ teaspoon ground cinnamon

Preheat oven to 350°F. Spray 2 baking sheets with vegetable spray.

With the back of a wooden spoon,
cream together butter and cheese in a
medium-size bowl. Add egg and mix in
well. Add skim milk, stirring to blend.
Mix in flour and cinnamon.

Fill pastry bag fitted with a large
star tip with dough. Pipe in 2-inch rounds
on prepared baking sheets and bake
each batch on middle shelf of oven until
golden, 12 to 15 minutes.

Remove to wire racks to cool.

Makes 24 cookies
(45 calories per cookie)

Skinny Piecrust

Rolling this dough out takes a little practice.

2 tablespoons butter
¼ cup whole wheat pastry
   flour

¼ cup unbleached white flour
4 to 8 teaspoons ice water

In a medium-size bowl, combine whole wheat pastry flour and unbleached white flour. Cut butter into flour with a pastry blender until crumbly. Add water, a teaspoon at a time, until dough clings together when pressed against the sides of the bowl. Form into a flat round, wrap in plastic wrap, and chill well.

Roll out lightly floured dough to paper thinness on cool surface between 2 pieces of waxed paper. Remove top piece of waxed paper.

For bottom crust only: Invert crust, paper side up, over pie plate. Remove second piece of paper and press crust against bottom and sides of plate. (There will be no ridge of crust as in a conventional pie.) To bake blind, prick bottom and sides with a fork and bake on bottom shelf of preheated 425°F oven until lightly browned, about 10 minutes.

For top crust only: Place crust over filling, paper side up. Remove second piece of paper. Press edges against edge of pie plate. Cut vents.

Makes 1 bottom or 1 top crust
(10   43-calorie servings)

Maple Pear Torte

1 recipe for Heavenly Angel Food
   Cake (page 42)
4 fresh pears
1½ teaspoons cornstarch
2 tablespoons maple syrup
½ teaspoon vanilla extract
1 cup Slim Pastry Cream
   (page 270)
16 pecan halves, optional

Bake angel food cake according to directions.

Halve, peel, and core pears. Place them cut side down in a large skillet. Cover with water. Cover pan and bring to a boil. Reduce heat and simmer for 5 minutes.

Remove pears with a slotted spoon and set them aside to cool.

Pour ⅓ cup of the liquid from pears into a small saucepan. Stir in cornstarch until it dissolves. Add maple syrup and heat, stirring constantly, until mixture thickens. Remove from heat, add vanilla, and set aside.

Cut cake in half crosswise. Place one layer on serving plate, reserving second layer for future use. Spread top with pastry cream. Arrange pears around edge, cut side down. Arrange pecan halves around pears, if desired. Drizzle maple glaze over pears and chill cake.

Makes 16 servings
(100 calories per serving)

Holiday Ice Cream Bombe

I use crumbs from Heavenly Angel Food Cake for this. But any cake crumbs will do.

3 cups French Carob Ice Milk
   (page 198), softened
½ cup Heavenly Angel Food Cake
   crumbs (page 42), divided
2½ cups Frozen Peach Brandy
   Supreme (page 126)
2 cups Banana Strawberry Freeze
   (page 120)
16 fresh strawberries

Line an 8-cup bombe mold with softened French Carob Ice Milk, pushing it against sides and leaving an even indentation in center. Sprinkle with ¼ cup cake crumbs. Cover mold with plastic wrap and freeze until firm, about 1 hour.

While French Carob Ice Milk is hardening, allow Frozen Peach Brandy to soften. Then form a layer of Frozen Peach Brandy inside the layer of French Carob Ice Milk, leaving an even indentation in center. Sprinkle with remaining cake crumbs. Cover mold with plastic wrap and freeze until firm, about 1 hour.

While Frozen Peach Brandy is hardening, allow Banana Strawberry Freeze to soften. Fill in indentation left in mold. Smooth top, cover with plastic wrap, and return to freezer until ready to serve.

To unmold, quickly dip bottom of mold in warm, not hot, water, and invert on a platter. Surround with strawberries.

Makes 15 servings
(119 calories per serving)

Tangy Banana Fluff

This tart, light dessert is ideal when you want a finale that's not too sweet.

1 envelope unflavored gelatin
1 cup freshly squeezed orange juice
3 tablespoons honey
1 cup plain low-fat yogurt
2 egg whites
⅛ teaspoon cream of tartar
1 medium-size ripe banana
6 mandarin orange sections, optional

In a small saucepan, sprinkle gelatin over orange juice. Set aside for 3 minutes to soften. Heat over low heat, stirring constantly, until gelatin dissolves. Remove from heat.

In a medium-size bowl, stir gelatin mixture, honey, and yogurt together. Chill until thickened but not set, stirring occasionally so edges won't set.

In a medium-size bowl, beat egg whites until foamy. Add cream of tartar and continue beating until stiff peaks form.

Cut banana into quarters, lengthwise. Cut quarters crosswise into small pieces. Fold into yogurt mixture. Fold in beaten egg whites and divide among 6 dessert glasses. Decorate with mandarin orange sections, if desired, and chill until set.

Makes 6 servings
(77 calories per serving)

Light Lemon Gelatin

⅓ cup freshly squeezed lemon juice
1½ cups water, divided
1 envelope unflavored gelatin
¼ cup honey
¼ teaspoon lemon extract
about 6 drops natural yellow food coloring

In a medium-size bowl, combine lemon juice and 1 cup of the water.

In a small saucepan, sprinkle gelatin over remaining water. Set aside to soften for 2 minutes. Add honey and heat over medium heat, stirring until gelatin dissolves. Add to juice mixture. Mix in lemon extract and food coloring and chill until set.

Makes 4 servings
(75 calories per serving)

Blueberry Rice Pudding

1¼ cups skim milk
  3 tablespoons honey
  2 eggs, beaten
1½ teaspoons vanilla extract
  1 teaspoon ground cinnamon
  2 cups cooked rice
  ¾ cup unsweetened frozen blue-
      berries, thawed

Preheat oven to 325°F. Spray a 1½-quart casserole with vegetable spray.

In a large bowl, whisk together skim milk, honey, eggs, vanilla, and cinnamon. Fold in rice and blueberries gently so berries won't break. Bake on middle shelf of oven until set near (but not in) center, 45 to 50 minutes.

Remove from oven and allow to cool slightly.

Makes 8 servings
(125 calories per serving)

Apple-Filled German Pancakes

The middle of this oven-cooked treat sinks and the edges rise as it bakes.

  3 eggs
  ½ cup skim milk
  2 teaspoons honey
  ¼ cup whole wheat pastry flour
  ¼ cup unbleached white flour
  1 cup Applesauce (page 90)
  ½ teaspoon ground cinnamon

Preheat oven to 425°F. Spray a 9-inch pie plate with vegetable spray.

In a medium-size bowl, beat eggs with a whisk until foamy. Beat in skim milk and honey.

In a small bowl, sift together whole wheat pastry flour and unbleached white flour, whisking to blend. Beat into egg mixture until just mixed. Pour into prepared pan and bake on middle shelf of oven until lightly browned, 15 to 20 minutes.

Remove from oven and fill indentation with Applesauce. Sprinkle with cinnamon, slice, and serve immediately.

Makes 8 servings
(83 calories per serving)

Mock Whipped Cream

This keeps well in the refrigerator for about a day.

1½ teaspoons unflavored
    gelatin
¼ cup boiling water
1½ teaspoons honey

1 cup ice water
½ cup instant nonfat dry milk
2 teaspoons vanilla extract

Chill a large bowl and beaters.
Dissolve gelatin in boiling water. Stir in honey.
In chilled bowl, beat together ice water, nonfat dry milk, and vanilla until very frothy. Gradually add gela-tin mixture and continue beating until quite stiff. Chill for at least 1 hour before using.

Makes about 4 cups
(3 calories per tablespoon)

Coffee Granita with Cream

The correct way to treat a granita is to freeze it until it's quite solid, then shave it into dessert dishes at serving time. But it can be served in scoops like a sherbet or ice.

1 quart boiling water
2 tablespoons decaffeinated
    instant coffee (3 if you want
    a strong coffee taste)
⅓ cup honey
½ cup Mock Whipped Cream
    (page 10), divided

In a medium-size bowl, mix together all ingredients except whipped cream and let mixture cool.
Process mixture in an ice cream maker according to manufacturer's instructions, or turn mixture into a large pan and freeze until thick but not solid. Remove from freezer, beat to break down ice crystals, and then return to freezer. Repeat this procedure twice.
At serving time top each portion with 1 tablespoon of the Mock Whipped Cream.

Makes 8 servings
(46 calories per serving)

Peachy Scallop

4 cups unsweetened frozen sliced
   peaches, thawed
2 tablespoons honey
1 teaspoon vanilla extract
¾ teaspoon ground cinnamon
¼ teaspoon ground nutmeg

Preheat oven to 350°F.
Mix peaches with other ingredients
in a 1½-quart casserole. Bake on middle
shelf of oven until peaches are tender,
about 20 minutes. Serve warm.

Makes 4 servings
(97 calories per serving)

Fruited Orange Cups

2 large oranges
½ cup unsweetened frozen
   cherries, thawed
½ cup unsweetened crushed
   pineapple
2 tablespoons raisins, plumped
8 seedless green grapes, quartered

Cut oranges into halves. Carefully
cut out pulp, leaving shells intact. Chop
orange pulp, removing seeds and pith.
Combine with remaining ingredients in
a medium-size bowl and chill to blend
flavors.
To serve, mound fruit in orange shells.

Makes 4 servings
(97 calories per serving)

Peanut Pear Pie

1 recipe for Skinny Piecrust
   (page 6)
5 cups peeled fresh pear chunks
3 tablespoons honey
2 tablespoons freshly squeezed
   lemon juice
2 tablespoons chopped raisins
2 tablespoons chopped peanuts
1 teaspoon ground cinnamon
1 tablespoon whole wheat pastry
   flour

Preheat oven to 400°F. Line a 9-inch
pie plate with pastry and bake blind according to directions.
In a large bowl, toss pears with remaining ingredients, mixing well. Turn
into prepared piecrust and bake on bottom shelf of oven until crust is golden
and fruit is tender, about 40 minutes.

Makes 10 servings
(130 calories per serving)

Easy Vanilla Frosting

1 egg white
¼ teaspoon cream of tartar
2 tablespoons honey

1 teaspoon vanilla extract
½ cup instant nonfat dry milk*

In a small bowl, beat egg white until foamy. Add cream of tartar and continue to beat, adding honey and vanilla. Gradually add nonfat dry milk, beating constantly.

Makes about 1 cup
(20 calories per tablespoon)

*Use a very fine-textured nonfat dry milk for this recipe.

Apple and Spice Cake

The sweeter and juicier the apples you select for this cake, the more delicious the finished product will be.

4 eggs
½ cup honey
½ cup vegetable oil
1½ teaspoons vanilla extract
¾ cup whole wheat pastry flour
¾ cup unbleached white flour
2 teaspoons baking powder
2 teaspoons ground cinnamon
½ teaspoon ground nutmeg
2 medium-size apples
1 cup Delicious Diet Cream
(page 119), divided
ground cinnamon for sprinkling

Preheat oven to 325°F. Spray a 9 × 9-inch pan with vegetable spray.

In a large bowl, beat together eggs, honey, oil, and vanilla.

Sift together whole wheat pastry flour, unbleached white flour, baking powder, cinnamon, and nutmeg and add to beaten ingredients. Mix together thoroughly.

Peel, core, and chop apples. Stir into batter and turn into prepared pan. Bake on middle shelf of oven until a cake tester inserted into center comes out clean, 30 to 35 minutes.

Serve warm or cold. Top each serving with a tablespoon of the diet cream and a sprinkle of cinnamon.

Makes 16 servings
(170 calories per serving)

Apple-Filled German Pancakes (page 9)

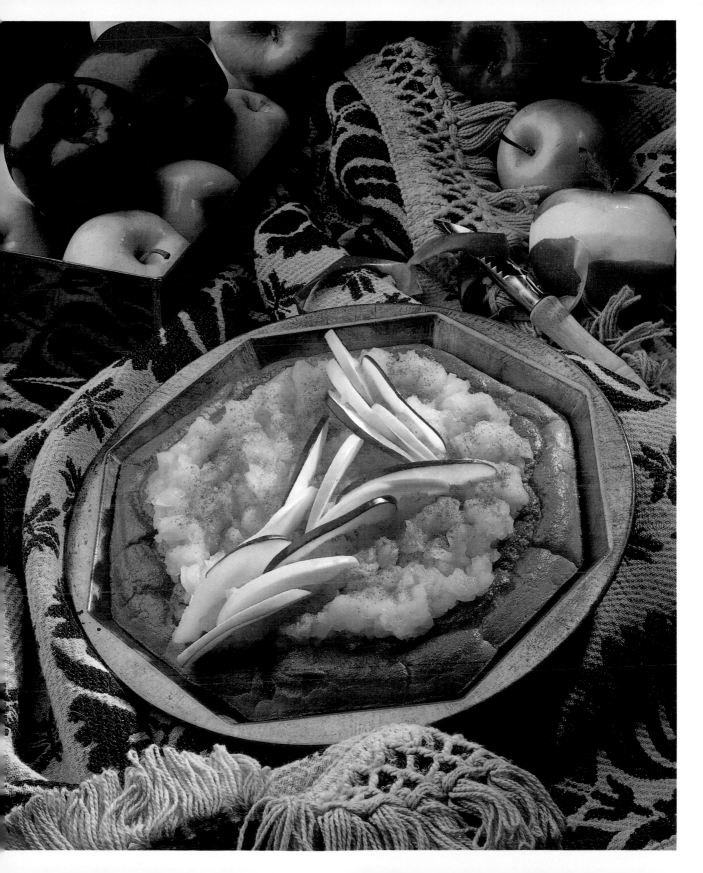

Apple Pear Bake

⅓ cup water
2 tablespoons freshly squeezed
   lemon juice
½ teaspoon ground ginger
1 teaspoon ground cinnamon
2 apples
2 fresh pears

Preheat oven to 350°F.

In a small bowl, mix together water, lemon juice, ginger, and cinnamon.

Peel and core apples and pears and cut into halves. Place in a casserole in a single layer. Pour water mixture over all, cover, and bake on middle shelf of oven until fruit is tender, about 30 minutes.

Put apple half and pear half in each of 4 dessert dishes.

Makes 4 servings
(99 calories per serving)

Jelly Shakes

4 envelopes unflavored gelatin
4 cups grape juice, divided

Sprinkle gelatin over 2 cups of the grape juice.

In a small saucepan, heat remaining juice to boiling. Add gelatin mixture and heat until gelatin dissolves, stirring constantly. Pour into a 9 × 13-inch pan and chill until set.

Cut into 1-inch squares.

Makes 117 squares
(6 calories per square)

Dream Pie

½ cup whole wheat pastry flour
½ cup unbleached white flour
1½ teaspoons baking powder
3 eggs
⅓ cup honey
1 teaspoon vanilla extract
¼ cup skim milk
1 cup Tangy Lemon Filling
   (page 244)
½ cup Easy Vanilla Frosting
   (page 12)

Preheat oven to 350°F. Spray 2 8-inch layer cake pans with vegetable spray.

Sift whole wheat pastry flour, unbleached white flour, and baking powder together into a small bowl.

In a large bowl, beat eggs until thick and light colored, about 7 minutes. Drizzle in honey and vanilla, beating for another minute.

Scald skim milk in a small pan.

Sift flour mixture into egg mixture, folding in. Add hot milk all at once, mixing in well. Turn batter into prepared pans and bake on middle shelf of oven until cake layers spring back when pressed lightly, 15 to 20 minutes.

Cool in pans inverted on wire racks.

Spread lemon filling on one cake layer. Place second layer on top and spread with vanilla frosting.

Makes 10 servings
(136 calories per serving)

Banana Coconut Ice Milk

    2 large, ripe bananas
    1 cup water
    1 cup skim milk
    ¼ cup nonfat dry milk
    3 tablespoons maple syrup
    2 teaspoons vanilla extract
    1 teaspoon lemon juice
    1 cup plain low-fat yogurt
    ½ cup unsweetened flaked coconut

Cut bananas into chunks. Puree in food processor. Add water, skim milk, nonfat dry milk, maple syrup, vanilla, and lemon juice, processing until smooth. Add yogurt and process just until blended.

Process mixture in an ice cream maker according to manufacturer's instructions. When processed, fold in coconut before putting in freezer. If you're not using an ice cream maker, turn mixture into a bowl and freeze until mushy. Remove from freezer, beat to break down ice crystals, and then return to freezer. Repeat this procedure twice, folding in coconut and spooning into a 1-quart, covered container the last time. Freeze until ready to serve.

Makes 8 servings
(86 calories per serving)

Peach Nut Bavarian

    1¼ cups skim milk
     2 eggs, separated
     2 envelopes unflavored gelatin
     ¼ cup honey
    1½ teaspoons vanilla extract
     ⅛ teaspoon cream of tartar
     ½ cup evaporated skim milk, chilled
     1 cup chopped unsweetened frozen peaches, thawed and well drained
     ¼ cup chopped walnuts

In the top of a double boiler, beat together skim milk and egg yolks. Sprinkle gelatin over mixture and allow to soften for 2 minutes. Add honey, set over hot, not boiling, water and cook, stirring constantly, until gelatin is dissolved. Remove from heat and mix in vanilla. Chill until thickened but not set, 25 to 30 minutes. Whisk briefly until smooth.

In a medium-size bowl, beat egg whites until foamy. Add cream of tartar and continue beating until stiff peaks form. Fold egg whites into gelatin mixture.

In a chilled, medium-size bowl, beat evaporated skim milk to the consistency of whipped cream. Fold peaches and nuts into gelatin mixture, then fold in whipped milk. Turn into a wet 8-cup mold and chill until set.

Unmold on platter at serving time.

Makes 12 servings
(78 calories per serving)

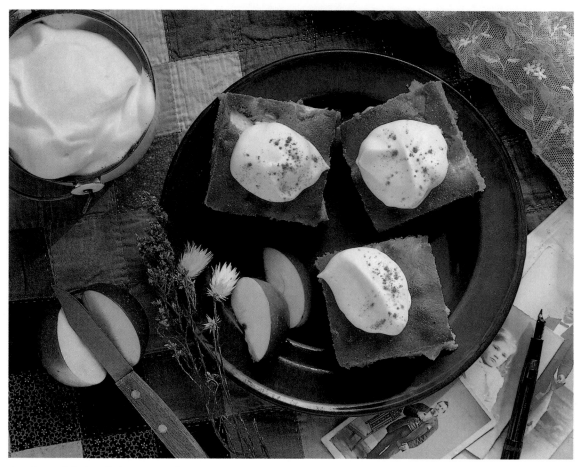

Apple and Spice Cake (page 12)

Mixed Fruit
with Raspberry Rum Sauce

12 seedless green grapes, divided
 2 ripe pears
 2 cups unsweetened frozen sliced
    peaches
½ teaspoon rum extract
 1 cup Ruby Raspberry Sauce
    (page 139)

Halve 8 grapes. Peel, core, and coarsely chop pears. Mix together grapes, pears, and peaches in a medium-size bowl.

Mix rum extract into raspberry sauce and toss with fruit. Divide among 4 dessert glasses. Decorate each with a whole grape.

Makes 4 servings
(113 calories per serving)

Coconut Thumb Prints

4 ounces low-fat creamed cottage
    cheese
6 tablespoons butter, softened
3 tablespoons honey
1 teaspoon vanilla extract
½ cup whole wheat pastry flour
½ cup unbleached white flour
⅓ cup Coconut Sugar (page 66)
    about 2 tablespoons red currant
    jelly, divided

In a food processor, process cheese, butter, honey, and vanilla.

In a large bowl, mix whole wheat pastry flour and unbleached white flour together with a wire whisk. With a wooden spoon, mix in cheese-butter mixture. Chill until firm enough to hold shape.

Spray 2 baking sheets with vegetable spray.

Preheat oven to 350°F.

Roll bits of dough (about 1 teaspoon) between palms of your hands into 1-inch balls. Roll balls in Coconut Sugar and place about 1 inch apart on prepared baking sheets, flattening slightly with back of spatula. With back of spoon, make a small indentation in each cookie. Put ⅛ teaspoon jelly in each indentation. Bake, 1 sheet at a time, on middle shelf of oven until coconut is lightly browned, 15 to 20 minutes.

Remove to wire racks to cool.

Makes 3 dozen cookies
(44 calories per cookie)

Strawberry French Toast

Usually thought of as breakfast fare, this version of French toast makes a marvelous dessert.

1 egg
½ cup skim milk
½ cup unsweetened frozen straw-
    berries, pureed
¼ teaspoon vanilla extract
4 slices whole grain bread
¼ cup Mock Whipped Cream
    (page 10), divided
4 whole unsweetened frozen
    strawberries, thawed, divided

Spray a large griddle with vegetable spray. Heat to medium.

In a medium-size bowl, beat egg. Whisk in skim milk, strawberry puree, and vanilla extract. Soak bread on both sides in mixture. Cook on griddle until lightly browned on both sides, turning once.

Serve each slice topped with 1 tablespoon of the Mock Whipped Cream and a strawberry.

Makes 4 servings
(100 calories per serving)

Coconut Crust

1½ cups unsweetened flaked
  coconut

1½ tablespoons butter,
  softened

Preheat oven to 325°F.
In a medium-size bowl, combine coconut and butter. Whirl briefly in a blender. Line a 9-inch pie plate with mixture and bake on middle shelf of oven until coconut is golden, about 15 minutes.

Cool before using. Crust will firm up as it cools.

Makes 1 piecrust
(8 65-calorie servings)

Mock Doughnut Holes

If you want these to look festive, add a drop or two of natural food coloring to the frosting.

reserved cut-out cake from
  Discovery Cake (page 221)
½ cup freshly made Easy Vanilla
  Frosting (page 12)
skim milk
⅓ cup Coconut Sugar (page 66)

Between the palms of your hands, lightly roll cake into 12 balls. Quickly roll each ball in frosting. (If frosting becomes too thick or stiff, work in just enough skim milk to make it loose.) Roll frosted balls in Coconut Sugar before frosting dries.

Makes 12 doughnut holes or 6 servings
(174 calories per serving)

Beautiful Baked Alaska

1 quart Raspberry Rum Sherbet
  (page 165), softened
1 Lazy Day Loaf Cake (page 201)
10 egg whites
¼ teaspoon cream of tartar
1 tablespoon honey
1½ teaspoons vanilla extract

Line a round 2-quart bowl with plastic wrap. Pack softened sherbet into it, smoothing top. Cover with plastic wrap and return to freezer until very firm.

Cut cake lengthwise into 4 pieces. Fit together side by side, and cut into a circle 1½ to 2 inches larger than the top of bowl containing sherbet. Place cake on baking sheet.

Unmold sherbet on top of cake. Cover and return to freezer until very firm.

Just before serving, preheat oven to 450°F.

In a large bowl, beat egg whites until foamy. Add cream of tartar and continue beating, drizzling in honey and vanilla, until stiff peaks form. Working quickly, frost sherbet and cake with meringue, making peaks of meringue. Bake on middle shelf of oven until meringue is golden, about 4 minutes. Serve immediately.

Makes 14 servings
(197 calories per serving)

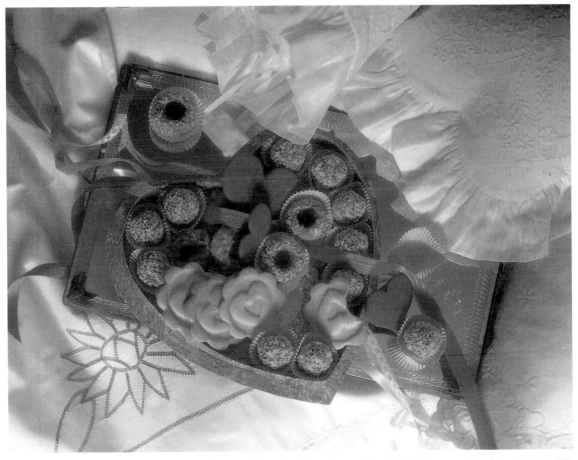

Coconut Thumb Prints (page 17)   Orange Date Cookies (page 70)   Light Lemon Cookies (page 133)
Molasses Ginger Joys (page 250)   Apricot Raisin Confections (page 268)

Apple-Grape Drink

½ cup unsweetened frozen white
    grape juice concentrate
1½ cups club soda
1   cup apple juice

Dissolve grape juice concentrate in club soda. Stir in apple juice and serve over crushed ice.

Makes 4 servings
(95 calories per serving)

Lite Surprise Pudding

3 cups Carob Chip Pudding
   (page 201), divided
8 Carob Thins (page 55)
½ cup Ruby Raspberry Sauce
   (page 139)

Put 1½ cups Carob Chip Pudding into a 2-quart casserole. Top with Carob Thins. Spread Raspberry Sauce over cookies. Top with remaining pudding and chill until serving time.

Makes 8 servings
(108 calories per serving)

Delectable Carob Cake

You don't have to bake all angel cakes in tube pans. This one is thin enough to cook evenly in a 9-inch springform pan.

⅓ cup whole wheat pastry flour
⅓ cup unbleached white flour
3 tablespoons carob powder
10 egg whites
¼ teaspoon cream of tartar
¼ cup honey
1 teaspoon vanilla extract

Preheat oven to 350°F.
Sift together whole wheat pastry flour, unbleached white flour, and carob powder 3 times. Re-measure to equal ⅔ cup plus 3 tablespoons.
In a large bowl, beat egg whites until foamy. Add cream of tartar and continue beating, drizzling in honey and vanilla, until stiff peaks form. Fold flour mixture gently into egg whites, turn into 9-inch springform pan and bake on bottom shelf of oven until top springs back when lightly pressed, 35 to 40 minutes.
Cool completely upside down. Cut with serrated knife.

Makes 12 servings
(51 calories per serving)

Grapefruit Orange Pie

The fruit for this pie should be well drained before it's added to the other ingredients.

  1 recipe for Coconut Crust
      (page 18)
¼ cup cornstarch
1¼ cups skim milk
⅓ cup honey
¾ cup freshly squeezed orange
      juice
½ cup fresh grapefruit sections
½ cup fresh seedless orange
      sections

Bake Coconut Crust according to directions. Cool.

In a medium-size saucepan, dissolve cornstarch in skim milk. Add honey and bring to a boil, stirring constantly, until thickened. Remove from heat and stir in orange juice. Heat again, stirring until thickened. Remove from heat and fold in fruit. Allow to cool, stirring occasionally. Turn into piecrust and chill well before serving.

*Makes 10 servings
(121 calories per serving)*

Pears with Raspberry Sauce

¾ cup water
  2 tablespoons honey
½ teaspoon vanilla extract
  8 medium-size fresh pears, peeled,
      halved, and cored
  1 cup Ruby Raspberry Sauce
      (page 139), divided

In a large saucepan, bring water and honey to a boil. Stir in vanilla. Add pears, cover, and reduce heat to simmer, cooking until pears are soft, 6 to 8 minutes.

Drain and chill pears. Divide pear halves among 8 bowls, placing sides with indentations up. Fill each indentation with 1 tablespoon of the raspberry sauce and serve immediately.

*Makes 8 servings
(114 calories per serving)*

Pears à la Crème

1½ teaspoons cornstarch
½ cup unsweetened pineapple
    juice
½ teaspoon ground cinnamon
2 tablespoons honey
2 fresh pears
1 cup evaporated skim milk,
    chilled

In a medium-size saucepan, dissolve cornstarch in pineapple juice. Stir in cinnamon and honey.

Peel, core, and coarsely chop pears. Add to saucepan and bring to a boil, stirring constantly. Reduce heat, cover, and let simmer until pears are fork tender, about 10 minutes. Remove from heat and chill.

Just before serving, beat evaporated skim milk in a medium-size bowl until soft peaks form. Fold in pear mixture. Turn into 8 dessert glasses and serve immediately.

Makes 8 servings
(73 calories per serving)

★ Apple Raisin Pie

1 recipe for Skinny Piecrust
    (page 6)
5 apples
½ cup raisins, plumped
1 teaspoon ground cinnamon
1 teaspoon vanilla extract
2 teaspoons freshly squeezed
    lemon juice
2 tablespoons cornstarch

Preheat oven to 425°F. Line a 9-inch pie plate with pastry according to directions. Chill.

Peel, core, and thinly slice apples into a bowl of cold water, to which 1 teaspoon of lemon juice has been added. Drain apple slices well and toss with remaining ingredients. Turn into prepared pie shell, cover with foil, and bake on bottom shelf of oven until crust is golden, 35 to 40 minutes.

Makes 10 servings
(110 calories per serving)

Easy Baked Pear Rings

4 **firm, ripe pears**
2 **tablespoons butter, melted**
2 **teaspoons honey**
   ground cinnamon for sprinkling

Preheat oven to 350°F. Spray a baking sheet with vegetable spray.

Peel, core, and slice pears into rounds about ½ inch thick. Arrange rounds on prepared baking sheet. In a small bowl, mix together butter and honey. Brush mixture on top of pear rings. Sprinkle with cinnamon and bake on middle shelf of oven for about 15 minutes, or until pears are fork tender.

Makes 6 servings
(108 calories per serving)

FEBRUARY

Spicing Up Desserts

				1	Ground Hog 2 Day	3
FRUIT OF THE MONTH: **BANANAS** *DESSERT OF THE MONTH:* **BANANA LEMON TORTE** *DRINK OF THE MONTH:* **TOMATO ZIP**				BANANA LEMON TORTE ★	FRIENDLY HERMITS	VERMONT PUDDING
4	5	6	7	8	9	10
CRUSTLESS COFFEE PIE	FRUITED DESSERT SHAKE	ORANGE SORBET	STRAWBERRY AMBROSIA	ROYAL RED TAPIOCA	PERFECT PEAR CREPES	FROZEN BANANA SQUARES
11	12	13	*Valentine's* 14 *Day*	15	16	17
GORGEOUS GRAPEFRUIT	UPSIDE-DOWN PINEAPPLE PIE	SWEET POTATO PUDDING	BE MY VALENTINE CAKE	AMERICAN APPLE BAKE	LEMON RAZMATAZ	BLACK AND WHITE PUDDING PIE
18	19	20	21	22	*Presidents'* 23 *Day*	24
ONE SMALL, RIPE BANANA	HEAVENLY ANGEL FOOD CAKE	BANANA PUDDING LAYERS	MOCK MOCHA POPS	CHEERY CHERRY PIE	PRESIDENTS' DAY PATRIOTIC PARFAITS	PFEFFERNUSSE
25	26	27	28	29		
FLUFFY BLUEBERRY OMELET	PEAR BREAD PUDDING	BANANA ROYAL	FROZEN STRAWBERRY FLUFF	FRUITY YOGURT PIE		

Fruity Yogurt Pie (page 45)

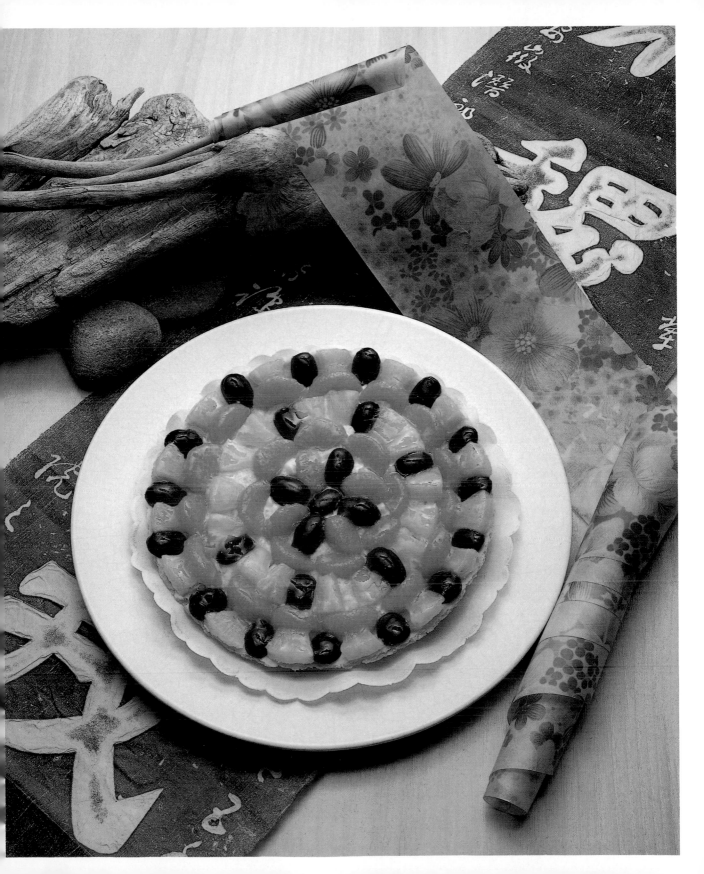

Spices and extracts are essential ingredients in many desserts, but their role is especially important in diet desserts where they are often relied upon to make up for the reduced sweetening that saves on calories. Vanilla is the single most useful essence for this. With a sweetness of its own, this quintessential extract can be used either as the primary flavoring or to bolster others.

Spices

Derived from the bark, leaves, seeds, stamens, fruit, flowers, or roots of a wide variety of tropical plants, spices come from faraway places with romantic names like the Spice Islands, Madagascar, and Zanzibar. In fact, allspice is the only commonly used spice native to the Western Hemisphere.

I don't use any hard-to-find spices in this book. Most desserts can be improved with the addition of such widely available spices as cinnamon, cloves, ginger, or nutmeg, although occasionally I do use allspice or anise seeds in a dessert.

Whole or Ground Spices

Whole spices, that you plan to grind yourself, will keep much longer than those already ground. Nutmeg is one spice most cooks use frequently that is considerably better when home-ground just prior to use. A small, readily available nutmeg grater will make this an easy chore.

When buying ground spices, don't be lured by large boxes at low prices. Ground spices don't become rancid, but they do lose their potency quickly and should therefore be purchased in very small quantities and used as soon as possible. Date each newly purchased container before storing it, and discard it after about six months. If you're not sure whether a spice has seen its day and should be thrown out, smell it. A musty odor means that the flavor is gone, and the container should be eliminated from your supply.

The spice section of any given market offers an array of spices sold in a variety of containers. Avoid those in cardboard boxes — the flavor leaches into the cardboard and is soon dissipated. And glass jars allow light, an enemy of freshness and long life for spices, into the containers. Select instead small tin boxes of ground spices.

Since both air and light rob spices of their freshness, get into the habit of closing a container immediately after you've measured the necessary amount.

Some cooks grind whole spices with a mortar and pestle. This is time consuming, and it produces a lumpy, uneven powder. The late James Beard, master chef and cookbook author, suggested the use of a small electric coffee mill to grind spices.

The best ground spices (other than home-ground) can be found in spice stores. If there aren't any in your region, you'll find that many sell spices mail order. Here are the names and addresses of a few companies that carry a large variety of spices:

Aphrodisia
282 Bleecker St.
New York, NY 10014
(212) 989-6440

Caprilands Herb Farm
534 Silver St.
Coventry, CT 06238
(203) 742-7244

Balducci's
424 Avenue of the Americas
New York, NY 10011
(212) 673-2600

While stylishly decorative spice shelves with a selection of jars of interesting shapes and sizes may add character to kitchens, they're not recommended for storing spices, as they leave them vulnerable to light and often stove heat. Keep spices secreted away in a cool, dark cabinet.

Spices must, of course, be added to cakes, pies, and cookies when you're making the batter or filling. But when you make pudding or any other loose-textured dessert in which it's possible to add a spice during the cooking process, do so. For best results, add spices about ten minutes before a dessert is finished cooking. The heat of cooking greatly diminishes the strength of spices.

Extracts

While lacking the romance of spices, extracts are nonetheless just as essential for dessert making. A dash of almond, a spoonful of vanilla, or a hint of mint can be either the featured flavoring or play a supporting, but important, role in the production of a dessert.

Spices and Some Other Flavorings for Diet Desserts

One of the most important aspects of making successful desserts is an understanding of flavorings. The following table suggests ways to use some of the best of them in preparing diet desserts.

Allspice	Flavor of cinnamon, cloves, and nutmeg	Cakes, pies, puddings
Almond	Strong, nutlike extract	Cakes, candies, cookies, pies, puddings
Anise seeds	Licorice taste	Candies, cookies
Cinnamon	Aromatic, tangy—very useful in diet desserts	Cakes, cookies, pies, puddings
Cloves	Pungent	Cakes, cookies, pies
Ginger	A bit hot and zesty	Candies, cakes, cookies, gingerbread, puddings
Lemon	Very tart extract	Cakes, cookies, fillings, pies, puddings
Nutmeg	Sharp, nutty—best when ground just prior to use	Cakes, custards, drinks, pies, puddings
Orange	Citrus extract	Cakes, cookies, fillings, frostings, pies, puddings
Vanilla	Sweetish extract	All desserts

Extracts add few calories, but they can make the difference between an uninteresting dessert and a shining success. They can virtually dictate the flavor of a dessert. Using almond extract, for instance, in a cake traditionally made with vanilla extract will make it taste totally different. The recipes can be identical except for that one small difference, but what a difference! Or a small amount of extract can be added to a recipe producing a subtle, but important, change in flavor.

There is a huge array of extracts. I liberally use those I like. In diet desserts, where the object is maximum flavor for minimum calories, they're indispensable. For instance, I may add orange extract to an orange pudding made with fresh orange juice because I want a more pronounced orange taste without the calories of more orange juice.

The extracts I use most, and which I always have on my shelf, are vanilla (which I do buy in a big bottle because I use it so frequently and in quite large amounts), lemon, orange, almond, rum, brandy, and peppermint. Like spices, extracts should be closed tightly immediately after use and kept in a cool, dark place. Brandy and rum extracts make it possible to present more exotic desserts featuring those flavors without adding either alcohol or an appreciable number of calories.

Vanilla works well in tandem with almost any other extract, and combining other extracts, such as lemon and almond, lemon and rum, or brandy and orange, also makes interesting flavorings.

Always buy pure vanilla. The synthetic, called vanillin, while cheaper and stronger, smells like vanilla but has a slightly bitter, off taste that doesn't duplicate the flavor of real vanilla.

Almond is the strongest extract I use, and should be used cautiously at about half the strength of other extracts.

Heat destroys extracts and cold dulls the taste buds to them. Add extracts to a recipe as late as possible (after cooking is through is best). And when making a frozen or chilled dessert, you may need what seems like an incredible amount of extract. I taste a frozen-type dessert before processing or freezing it. When it tastes just about right, I add the same amount of extract that I've already used. Although the flavor is certainly powerful before the dessert is frozen, it turns out to be perfect after processing.

Friendly Hermits

A low-calorie version of an old favorite!

- ¼ cup raisins
- 5 tablespoons butter
- ⅓ cup honey
- 2 eggs
- ½ cup plain low-fat yogurt
- ½ cup whole wheat flour
- ½ cup unbleached white flour, divided
- ⅓ cup rolled oats
- 1 teaspoon ground cinnamon
- ½ teaspoon ground ginger
- ½ teaspoon baking powder

Cover raisins with warm water and set aside to plump.

Preheat oven to 350°F. Spray 2 baking sheets with vegetable spray.

In a large bowl, beat butter and honey together until fluffy. Beat in eggs. Fold in yogurt.

In a medium-size bowl, mix together whole wheat flour, ¼ cup of the unbleached white flour, oats, cinnamon, ginger, and baking powder, whisking to blend. Mix gently but thoroughly into moist ingredients.

Drain raisins well, and toss with remaining unbleached white flour. Fold into batter and drop batter by heaping teaspoonfuls onto 1 prepared baking sheet, pulling spoon along each mound of dough to make long cookies. Bake on middle shelf of oven until lightly browned, 15 to 18 minutes. While first batch is baking, repeat process with remaining dough.

Cool cookies on wire racks.

Makes 3 dozen cookies
(49 calories per cookie)

Crustless Coffee Pie

- 1 envelope unflavored gelatin
- ½ cup cold water
- 3 tablespoons honey
- ¾ teaspoon ground cinnamon, divided
- 2 teaspoons vanilla extract
- 1 cup strong, hot decaffeinated coffee
- 3 eggs, separated
- ⅛ teaspoon cream of tartar

Spray a 9-inch pie plate with vegetable spray.

In a small saucepan, sprinkle gelatin over cold water. Set aside for 5 minutes to soften.

Stir in honey, ¼ teaspoon of the cinnamon, and vanilla into coffee. Set aside.

In the top of a double boiler set over hot, not boiling, water, beat egg yolks until slightly thickened, about 3 minutes. Gradually stir in coffee mixture. Remove from heat.

Heat gelatin mixture over medium heat, stirring constantly, until gelatin dissolves. Whisk into coffee mixture. Chill until slightly thickened.

In a medium-size bowl, beat egg whites until foamy. Add cream of tartar and continue to beat until stiff peaks form. Fold coffee mixture into egg whites. Turn into prepared pie plate, sprinkle with remaining cinnamon, and chill until set.

Makes 8 servings
(58 calories per serving)

Banana Lemon Torte

1 recipe for Pretty Peach Layer
   Cake (page 128)
1 envelope unflavored gelatin
¾ cup water
2 tablespoons honey
¼ cup freshly squeezed lemon juice
   natural yellow food coloring
1 ripe banana

Bake cake according to directions.

In a small saucepan, sprinkle gelatin over water. Set aside to soften for 5 minutes. Heat, over medium heat, stirring constantly, until gelatin dissolves. Remove from heat and stir in honey and lemon juice. Add a few drops of food coloring. Chill, stirring often, until mixture is thickened but not set.

Wrap and freeze 1 layer of the cake for future use. Place the second layer on a serving plate. Slice banana. Arrange slices on top of cake. Spread gelatin mixture over fruit and chill until set.

Makes 12 servings
(63 calories per serving)

Vermont Pudding

1 envelope unflavored gelatin
½ cup cold water
¼ cup plus 1 tablespoon maple
   syrup, divided
1 teaspoon vanilla extract
1 cup evaporated milk, chilled
1 egg white
⅛ teaspoon cream of tartar
2 tablespoons grape-nuts cereal,
   divided

In a small saucepan, sprinkle gelatin over cold water. Set aside for 5 minutes to soften. Stir in ¼ cup maple syrup. Heat over medium heat, stirring constantly, until gelatin dissolves. Remove from heat and stir in vanilla and evaporated milk. Put in large bowl and chill until slightly thickened.

In a small bowl, beat egg white until foamy. Add cream of tartar and beat until stiff peaks form.

Beat gelatin mixture to the consistency of whipped cream. Fold in egg white and divide among 6 dessert glasses. Sprinkle 1 teaspoon grape-nuts over each pudding. Drizzle ½ teaspoon maple syrup over top. Refrigerate until serving time.

Makes 6 servings
(91 calories per serving)

Fruited Dessert Shake

½ cup unsweetened pineapple juice
½ cup freshly squeezed orange
    juice
½ cup skim milk
½ cup Vanilla Ice Milk (page 79)

In a blender, whirl together pineapple juice, orange juice, skim milk, and Vanilla Ice Milk. Divide between 2 glasses and serve at once.

Makes 2 servings
(144 calories per serving)

Royal Red Tapioca

1¼ cups red grape juice
1¼ cups water
  2 tablespoons honey
 ¼ cup quick-cooking tapioca
  1 teaspoon vanilla extract

In a medium-size saucepan, combine all ingredients. Set aside for 5 minutes to soften tapioca.
Bring to a boil over medium heat, stirring occasionally. Allow to boil 1 minute, stirring constantly. Chill.

Makes 6 servings
(76 calories per serving)

Strawberry Ambrosia

2 seedless oranges, chopped
1 pink seedless grapefruit,
   chopped
½ cup seedless green or red
   grapes, halved
1 cup unsweetened frozen
   strawberries, thawed
1 cup unsweetened flaked coconut
¼ cup freshly squeezed orange
   juice
1 teaspoon freshly squeezed
   lemon juice
1 banana

In a large bowl, combine all ingredients except banana and toss well. Slice banana, add to fruit mixture, and toss again.

Makes 10 servings
(74 calories per serving)

Delicious Diet Crepes

These crepes can be frozen by putting waxed paper between each crepe and wrapping all with plastic wrap, then foil.

2 eggs
1 teaspoon honey
⅔ cup skim milk
1¼ cups water
½ cup whole wheat pastry flour

½ cup unbleached white flour
½ teaspoon baking powder
½ teaspoon vanilla extract

In a large bowl, beat together eggs and honey. Beat in skim milk and water.

Sift together whole wheat pastry flour, unbleached white flour, and baking powder. Stir into egg mixture just until blended. Stir in vanilla. Cover and let mixture stand in refrigerator for at least 1 hour.

Spray an 8-inch skillet with vegetable spray. Heat over medium heat until a drop of water dropped in the middle of the skillet sizzles. Pour ⅛ cup of batter into pan, moving pan from side to side to distribute it evenly. When bubbles form on surface, about 45 seconds, turn crepe over and cook another 15 seconds. Repeat process until batter is finished.

Makes 16 crepes
(43 calories per crepe)

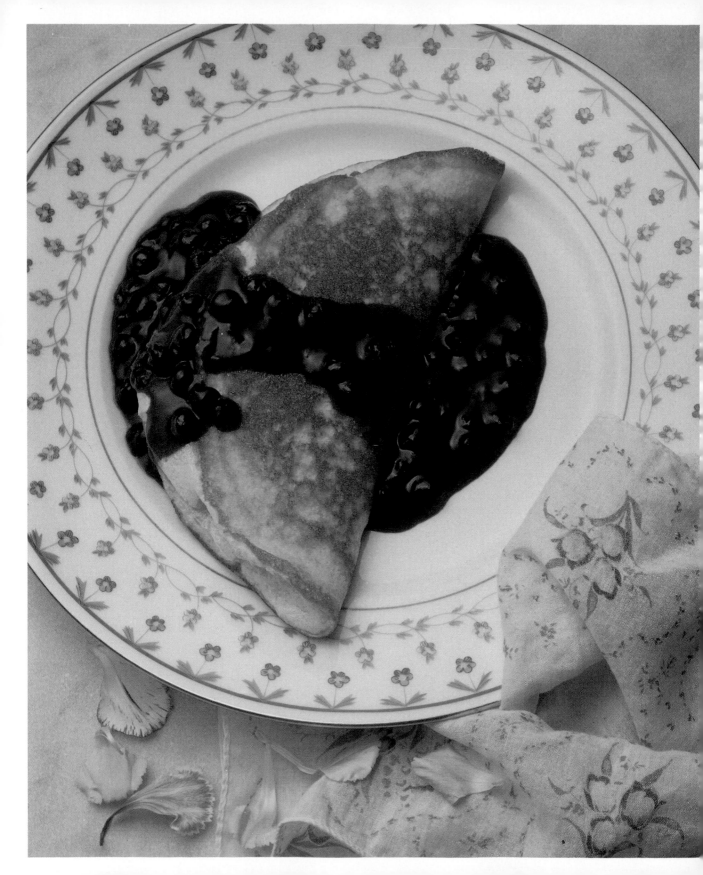

Be My Valentine Cake

⅓ cup whole wheat pastry flour
¼ teaspoon baking powder
1 egg white
1 egg, separated
⅛ teaspoon cream of tartar
2 tablespoons cold water
3 tablespoons honey
½ teaspoon almond extract
1 teaspoon vanilla extract
natural red food coloring
½ cup Decorator Frosting
(page 38)

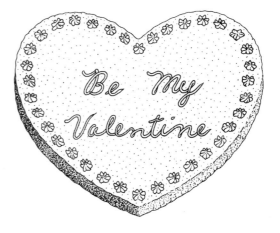

Preheat oven to 325°F. Line bottom of a heart-shaped 8-inch cake pan with waxed paper cut out in heart shape.

Sift together flour and baking powder into a small bowl. Whisk to blend.

In a medium-size bowl, beat egg whites until foamy. Add cream of tartar and continue beating until stiff peaks form.

In a large bowl, beat together egg yolk and water until foamy. Add honey and extracts and continue beating for 8 minutes. Fold in flour mixture, then beaten egg whites. Turn into prepared pan and bake on middle shelf of oven for 30 minutes.

Run a knife around edges of pan and turn out onto a wire rack. Remove waxed paper and allow to cool before decorating.

Add natural red food coloring to Decorator Frosting. Make stars around edge of cake with star tip. Write on top of cake with writing tip.

Makes 6 servings
(158 calories per serving)

Perfect Pear Crepes

2 cups diced fresh pears
2 teaspoons honey
¼ teaspoon ground cinnamon
⅛ teaspoon ground nutmeg
2 tablespoons ground pecans
8 Delicious Diet Crepes (page 33)
½ cup plain nonfat yogurt, divided

In a blender, puree pears. Turn into a medium-size saucepan. Add honey, cinnamon, and nutmeg and cook over medium heat, stirring constantly, for 5 minutes. Stir in nuts.

Divide among crepes, spooning mixture in a line down the middle of each one. Roll first 1 side over filling, then the other side. Spoon 1 tablespoon of the yogurt on top of each crepe and serve immediately.

Makes 8 servings
(84 calories per serving)

Fluffy Blueberry Omelet (page 46)

Upside-Down Pineapple Pie

1 20-ounce can unsweetened
      crushed pineapple
1 cup part-skim ricotta cheese
2 eggs
2 tablespoons honey
2 teaspoons vanilla extract

Preheat oven to 325°F. Spray a 10-inch pie plate with vegetable spray.

Drain pineapple thoroughly, reserving juice.

In a blender or food processor, combine reserved juice, ricotta, eggs, honey, and vanilla.

Spread crushed pineapple in prepared pie plate. Pour blended ingredients over pineapple and bake on middle shelf of oven for 50 to 60 minutes, or until a knife inserted near the center comes out clean. Serve warm or chilled.

Makes 12 servings
(43 calories per serving)

Frozen Banana Squares

2 very ripe bananas
1 cup part-skim ricotta cheese
2 tablespoons honey
1 teaspoon vanilla extract
¾ cup evaporated skim milk,
      chilled

In a food processor, puree bananas and ricotta. Add honey and vanilla.

In a large bowl, beat evaporated skim milk to the consistency of whipped cream. Fold in banana mixture. Turn into an 8 × 8-inch pan, cover, and freeze. Cut into 16 2-inch squares. Allow to soften slightly before serving.

Makes 16 squares
(32 calories per square)

Gorgeous Grapefruit

2 seedless pink grapefruits
2 egg whites
⅛ teaspoon cream of tartar
¼ teaspoon vanilla extract
4 fresh sweet cherries, pitted

Preheat oven to 350°F.

Cut grapefruits into halves. Run serrated knife between skins and pulp, then run knife between membranes and pulp, loosening sections.

In a medium-size bowl, beat egg whites until foamy. Add cream of tartar and vanilla and continue to beat until stiff peaks form. Divide evenly and pile on top of halved grapefruits, bringing beaten egg whites to edges of fruit. Place in a pan and bake on middle shelf of oven 12 to 15 minutes, or until meringue browns.

Cool and top each meringue with a cherry.

Makes 4 servings
(53 calories per serving)

Black and White Pudding Pie

1 recipe for Skinny Piecrust
  (page 6)
1 cup Very Vanilla Pudding
  (page 84)
1 cup Creamy Carob Pudding
  (page 176)
2 tablespoons ground walnuts,
  optional

Line a 9-inch pie plate with pastry and bake according to directions. Allow to cool thoroughly.

Spread cooled vanilla pudding in pie shell. Top with a layer of cooled carob pudding, spreading it to cover vanilla pudding. Sprinkle with nuts, if desired, and refrigerate until serving time.

Makes 8 servings
(124 calories per serving)

Decorator Frosting

This frosting must be used as soon as it is made. However, if you're using frosting in several colors, you can quickly put each color in a plastic decorating bag, folding down the top to prevent exposure to the air. If the frosting gets too hard, try beating in a bit of skim milk—a few drops at a time. Only fine-textured dry milk will work for this recipe!

2 egg whites
½ teaspoon cream of tartar
3 tablespoons honey
2 teaspoons vanilla extract

2 cups instant nonfat dry milk
natural food coloring, optional

In a medium-size bowl, beat egg whites until foamy. Beat in cream of tartar, honey, and vanilla. Slowly add nonfat dry milk, beating until stiff and glossy. If you're using food coloring, beat in a few drops until you reach desired shade.

Makes about 1¼ cups
(49 calories per tablespoon)

Banana Pudding Layers

3 cups Very Vanilla Pudding
  (page 84), divided
12 Light Lemon Cookies (page 133),
  divided
1 ripe banana, divided

Put 1 cup of the pudding into a 1½-quart casserole. Top with 6 cookies. Thinly slice banana and put half of the slices on top of cookies. Top with 1 cup of the pudding, the remaining cookies, and the rest of the banana slices. Spread remaining pudding on top and chill until serving time.

Makes 8 servings
(163 calories per serving)

Mock Mocha Pops

3 tablespoons Versatile Carob Syrup
  (page 162)
1 tablespoon strong decaffeinated
  coffee
1 envelope unflavored gelatin
2 cups water
2 tablespoons honey

In a small saucepan, combine carob syrup and coffee. Sprinkle gelatin over mixture and set aside for 5 minutes to soften. Add water and heat over medium heat, stirring constantly, until gelatin dissolves. Add honey. Pour into 8 2-ounce pop molds and freeze until very firm.

Makes 8 pops
(24 calories per pop)

American Apple Bake

4 baking apples
¼ cup water
1 teaspoon freshly squeezed
  lemon juice
2 tablespoons honey, warmed
¼ teaspoon ground nutmeg
½ cup grated cheddar cheese
1 tablespoon whole wheat pastry
  flour
½ teaspoon ground cinnamon

Preheat oven to 350°F.
Peel, core, and slice apples. Turn into an 8 × 8-inch baking dish.
In a small bowl, combine water, lemon juice, honey, and nutmeg. Drizzle over apples. Cover and bake on middle shelf of oven until apples are fork tender, about 40 minutes.
In a medium-size bowl, toss together cheese, flour, and cinnamon. Sprinkle over apple slices. Return, uncovered, to oven until cheese melts, about 4 minutes.

Makes 8 servings
(95 calories per serving)

Lemon Razzmatazz

½ cup freshly squeezed lemon
    juice, strained
1½ cups water
1 10-ounce package unsweetened
    frozen raspberries, thawed
1½ envelopes unflavored gelatin
¼ cup honey
¼ teaspoon lemon extract

In a medium-size bowl, mix together lemon juice and water.

Drain raspberries, reserving juice. Strain reserved juice into a small saucepan. Sprinkle gelatin over top and set aside to soften for 2 minutes. Add honey and heat over medium heat, stirring constantly, until gelatin dissolves. Remove from heat, mix in lemon extract, and stir into lemon juice in bowl. Chill until thickened but not set, about 45 minutes. Fold in raspberries and turn into 6 decorative molds or 6 dessert glasses. Chill until set.

If using decorative molds, dip bottoms in warm water for about 30 seconds and unmold before serving.

Makes 6 servings
(99 calories per serving)

Sweet Potato Pudding

1 pound sweet potatoes
⅓ cup skim milk
3 tablespoons honey
1 teaspoon vanilla extract
1 teaspoon ground cinnamon
6 tablespoons unsweetened pine-
    apple juice, divided
3 tablespoons Coconut Sugar
    (page 66), divided

Peel and quarter sweet potatoes. In a medium-size saucepan, cook sweet potatoes in enough boiling water to cover until tender, about 20 minutes.

In a food processor, puree sweet potatoes with skim milk, honey, vanilla, and cinnamon. Divide among 6 dessert glasses. Top each with 1 tablespoon of the pineapple juice and ½ tablespoon of the Coconut Sugar. Serve immediately.

Makes 6 servings
(123 calories per serving)

Presidents' Day Patriotic Parfaits

This recipe is a tribute to George and Abe as well as all our other presidents — past and present.

1½ cups skim milk
¼ cup honey
2 egg yolks, beaten
1 envelope unflavored gelatin
1 teaspoon vanilla extract
16 ounces part-skim ricotta cheese
1½ cups unsweetened frozen blueberries, thawed, divided
1½ cups unsweetened frozen raspberries, thawed, divided

In a medium-size saucepan, beat together skim milk, honey, and egg yolks. Sprinkle gelatin over top and set aside for 5 minutes to soften. Heat over low heat, whisking constantly, until gelatin dissolves, about 5 minutes. Mix in vanilla.

In a large bowl, beat ricotta until smooth. Beat in gelatin mixture and chill, stirring occasionally, until thick but not set.

Put a layer of cheese mixture in each of 6 parfait glasses. Top with 2 tablespoons of the blueberries. Add another layer of cheese mixture. Top with 2 tablespoons of the raspberries, another layer of cheese, 2 tablespoons of the blueberries, another layer of cheese, and end with 2 tablespoons of the raspberries. Chill until cheese is set.

Makes 6 servings
(193 calories per serving)

Cheery Cherry Pie

3¾ cups unsweetened frozen cherries
¼ cup raisins, plumped
¼ cup honey
1 tablespoon cornstarch
¼ cup water
1 teaspoon brandy extract
1 recipe for Mini Piecrust (page 113)

In a large saucepan, toss cherries, raisins, and honey together.

Dissolve cornstarch in water and stir into cherry mixture. Cook over medium heat, stirring constantly, until mixture thickens. Remove from heat and add brandy extract. Set aside for 15 minutes.

Preheat oven to 400°F. Line a 9-inch pie plate with Mini Piecrust according to directions. Turn cherry mixture into prepared piecrust. Cover with foil tent and bake on bottom shelf of oven until crust is lightly browned, 50 to 60 minutes.

Makes 10 servings
(130 calories per serving)

Heavenly Angel Food Cake

The only trick to making this easy cake is in folding in the flour. To keep the air in the batter, never let the spoon or spatula emerge from the batter during the folding process.

10 egg whites
 1 teaspoon cream of tartar
⅔ cup honey
½ cup whole wheat pastry flour
½ cup unbleached white flour
 2 teaspoons vanilla extract

Preheat oven to 350°F.

In a large bowl, beat egg whites until foamy. Add cream of tartar and beat until stiff peaks form. Drizzle in honey, beating just to blend.

Sift whole wheat pastry flour and unbleached white flour together 3 times. Measure 1 cup and sprinkle it on top of beaten egg whites. Fold flour in thoroughly but gently. Fold in vanilla extract. Pour batter into a 10-inch tube pan with removable tube and bake for 35 to 40 minutes, or until top springs back when lightly pressed with fingertips.

Invert pan on a wire rack until cake is completely cool. Run a knife around edges and turn out onto plate. Run knife along bottom to release tube.

Makes 16 servings
(87 calories per serving)

Pear Bread Pudding

 4 slices whole grain bread
1½ cups skim milk
 2 tablespoons honey
 3 eggs
½ teaspoon ground cinnamon
¼ teaspoon ground nutmeg
 2 pears
¼ cup raisins, plumped

Preheat oven to 325°F. Spray a 2-quart casserole with vegetable spray.

Toast bread and cut into cubes.

In a medium-size saucepan, scald skim milk. Remove from heat, add toast cubes and honey, and set aside briefly until toast is saturated.

In a medium-size bowl, beat together eggs, cinnamon, and nutmeg. Peel, core, and dice pears. Add, along with raisins, to egg mixture. Stir in bread and milk and turn into prepared casserole. Bake on middle shelf of oven until set, about 45 minutes.

Makes 6 servings
(177 calories per serving)

Presidents' Day Patriotic Parfaits (page 41)

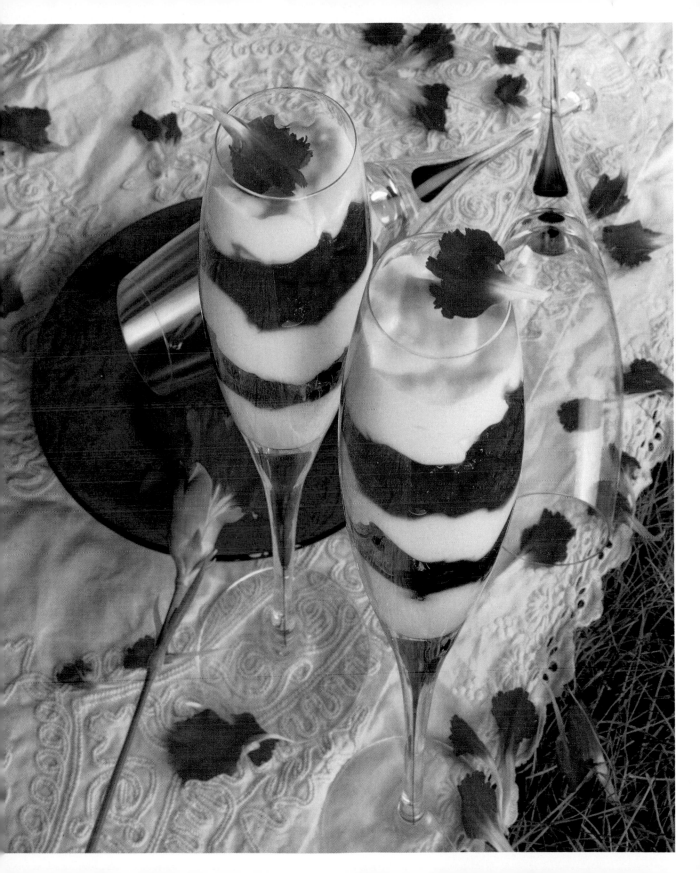

Pfeffernusse

This is a calorie-trimmed version of the traditional German Pepper Nut. It can be sliced into 1-inch rounds or cut with a small, decorative cookie cutter.

    1¼ cups whole wheat pastry flour
    1¼ cups unbleached white flour
     1 teaspoon ground cinnamon
     ½ teaspoon ground nutmeg
     ¼ teaspoon ground cloves
     ¼ teaspoon white pepper
     3 eggs
     ⅓ cup honey
     ½ teaspoon anise extract or
            1 teaspoon vanilla extract
     ⅓ cup walnuts
     ½ cup raisins

In a medium-size bowl, combine whole wheat pastry flour, unbleached white flour, cinnamon, nutmeg, cloves, and pepper, whisking to blend.

In a large bowl, beat eggs until foamy. Drizzle in honey and continue beating until very thick, about 8 minutes. Beat in extract.

In a food processor, finely chop walnuts and raisins with ¼ cup of flour mixture to keep raisins from sticking together. Mix into flour.

Stir flour-raisin mixture into eggs, blending well. Roll dough into a ball, wrap in plastic wrap, and chill until firm enough to roll.

Preheat oven to 325°F. Line 2 baking sheets with parchment paper.

Roll out one quarter of the dough between 2 pieces of waxed paper. Cut into desired shapes and place on pre-

pared baking sheets. Repeat process with remaining dough, one quarter at a time. Bake, 1 sheet at a time, on middle shelf of oven until firm, about 15 minutes. Remove to wire racks to cool.

The texture of these cookies will improve if you store them a day or 2 with a piece of bread in a tightly sealed container.

Makes 3 dozen cookies
(61 calories per cookie)

Tomato Zip

    6 ounces tomato juice
    2 drops Tabasco sauce
       wedge of lime

Mix together tomato juice and Tabasco in a small bowl. Squeeze a few drops of lime juice into mixture. Pour over ice in a glass and garnish with lime wedge.

Makes 1 serving
(35 calories per serving)

Fruity Yogurt Pie

1 recipe for Skinny Piecrust
    (page 6)
1 8-ounce can unsweetened
    pineapple chunks
1 envelope unflavored gelatin
1½ teaspoons vanilla extract
½ teaspoon ground cinnamon
½ cup plain low-fat yogurt
1¼ cups seedless red grapes,
    halved
1 cup mandarin orange sections

Line a 9-inch pie plate with pastry and bake blind according to directions. Cool.

Drain pineapple, reserving juice. Add enough water to juice to make 1¼ cups and transfer to small saucepan. Sprinkle gelatin over juice and set aside for 5 minutes to soften. Cook over medium heat, stirring constantly until gelatin dissolves. Remove 3 tablespoons of gelatin mixture and set aside. Add vanilla and cinnamon to remaining gelatin, mixing well, and chill until mixture reaches the consistency of egg whites, about 30 minutes.

Fold chilled gelatin into yogurt and turn into prepared piecrust. Chill about 15 minutes to set slightly. Arrange pineapple chunks, grapes, and orange sections on top of yogurt. Brush with reserved gelatin mixture, heating it briefly if it has thickened too much to brush on easily. Cover lightly with plastic wrap and chill until set.

Makes 10 servings
(77 calories per serving)

Frozen Strawberry Fluff

1 cup unsweetened frozen straw-
    berries, thawed
1 tablespoon honey
2 egg whites, at room temperature
½ cup evaporated skim milk,
    chilled

In a food processor, puree strawberries with honey.

In a medium-size bowl, beat evaporated skim milk to the consistency of whipped cream.

In a large bowl, beat egg whites until stiff peaks form. Fold beaten milk and then strawberry puree into egg whites. Freeze until ready to serve.

Makes 4 servings
(63 calories per serving)

Fluffy Blueberry Omelet

Folding in beaten egg whites makes this dessert omelet as light as air.

2 teaspoons cornstarch
½ cup freshly squeezed orange juice
½ cup unsweetened frozen blue-
     berries, thawed
2 tablespoons honey, divided
2 teaspoons vanilla extract
2 eggs, separated
2 eggs
⅛ teaspoon cream of tartar

In a jar with a tight-fitting lid, shake together cornstarch and orange juice.

In a small saucepan, mix together blueberries, orange juice mixture, and 1 tablespoon of the honey. Mash berries slightly with a fork to release juice. Simmer over medium heat, stirring constantly, until mixture thickens. Remove from heat. Stir in 1 teaspoon of the vanilla extract and set aside in a warm place.

In a medium-size bowl, beat egg yolks and whole eggs. Beat in remaining honey and vanilla.

In a large bowl, beat egg whites until foamy. Add cream of tartar and continue to beat until stiff peaks form. Fold egg yolks into egg whites.

Spray bottom and sides of a large nonstick skillet with vegetable spray. Heat over medium heat. Pour in egg mixture and cook over medium heat for about 2 minutes. Cover and cook 2 minutes more. Remove from heat.

Spread half of warm blueberry mixture on half of cooked omelet. Fold other half over. Remove to warmed platter and pour remaining sauce over top.

Makes 6 servings
(97 calories per serving)

Orange Sorbet

2 cups freshly squeezed orange
     juice
2 cups water, divided
3 tablespoons honey
1 teaspoon orange extract

Strain orange juice into a large bowl. Add 1½ cups of the water. In a small saucepan, heat remaining water and honey until honey dissolves. Pour into large bowl. Add extract and mix well.

Process mixture in an ice cream maker according to manufacturer's instructions, or turn mixture into a large pan and place in freezer until mushy. Remove from freezer, beat to break down ice crystals, and then return to freezer. Repeat this procedure twice. Freeze until ready to serve.

Makes about 10 servings
(42 calories per serving)

Banana Royal

1 cup freshly squeezed orange
    juice
1 cup water, divided
1 envelope unflavored gelatin
1 tablespoon honey
¼ teaspoon orange extract
1 ripe banana
½ cup seedless red grapes, halved

In a medium-size bowl, mix together orange juice and ½ cup of the water.

In a medium-size saucepan, sprinkle gelatin over remaining water. Set aside for 5 minutes to soften. Add honey and heat over medium heat, stirring constantly, until gelatin dissolves. Add to juice. Mix in orange extract and chill until thickened but not set.

Chop banana and fold into gelatin. Fold in grape halves and chill until set.

Makes 7 servings
(49 calories per serving)

MARCH

Beverages to Diet With

		1	2	3
FRUIT OF THE MONTH: **ORANGES** DESSERT OF THE MONTH: **ORANGE MERINGUE CUPS** DRINK OF THE MONTH: **GRAPE FIZZ**		CAKE ROLL PRUNEAU	PINEAPPLE CHARLOTTE	CAROB THINS
4 LUSCIOUS CITRUS PIE	5 RAISIN PEAR BREAD PUDDING	6 ORANGE MERINGUE CUPS ★	7 CAROB CHIPPERS	8 FROZEN PUDDING	9 PEANUT BUTTER APPLES	10 BANANA CREAM PIE
11 INDIVIDUAL STRAWBERRY CHEESE PUDDINGS	12 RING OF PLENTY	13 LUSCIOUS LEMON CHEESCAKE	14 SPICY PEARS	15 HAWAIIAN SNOW BALLS	16 SQUASH CUSTARD	*Saint Patrick's Day* 17 SAINT PADDY'S DAY MINT TREAT
18 ALMOND COCONUT CHIFFON PIE	19 ONE SMALL ORANGE, PEELED AND SECTIONED	20 BRANDY ZABAGLIONE	21 SUPER SPICE CAKE	22 STUFFED BAKED PEARS	23 ORANGE DATE COOKIES	24 NICE SPICE POPCORN
25 TANGY TANGERINE CREPES	26 BAKED JUNGLE TREAT	27 CAROB CHIP PIE	28 LEMON SORBET	29 LIGHT CARROT CAKE	30 RUM-TUM-DIDDLE SOUFFLÉS	31 TANGERINE BREAD PUDDING WITH PEACH SAUCE

Ring of Plenty (page 61)

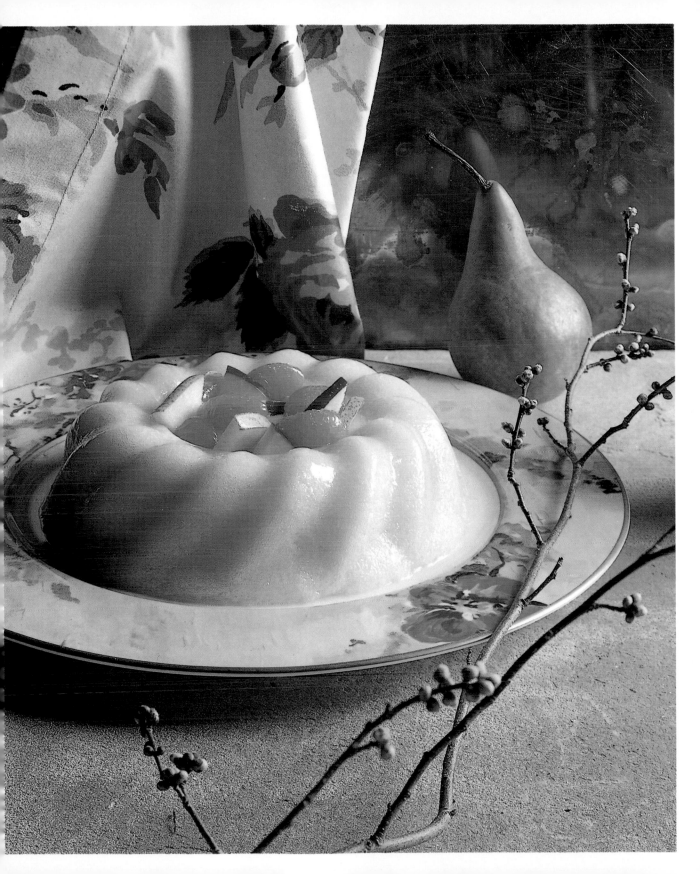

Water is, of course, the perfect beverage. I always keep a large pitcher of it in my refrigerator—nothing is quite as thirst-quenching. Whether you're dieting or not, you should drink six to eight glasses of this no-calorie super drink every day. Water, like all beverages, tends to make you feel full, so it's an effective alternative to food when you're hungry and know you shouldn't be eating. To make water especially appealing, serve it over ice cubes or crushed ice with a slice of lemon floating in each glass.

Coffee, without milk or sweetener, has only four calories a cup, and plain tea has no calories, so they are options for the dieter. But while the calorie count is tempting, the caffeine both contain isn't. I use decaffeinated coffee and herbal teas.

One of my favorite all-weather drinks is club soda. I find it's an exhilarating pick-me-up alone or when a few drops of lemon juice are added, and a great base for all types of fruit drinks. It's calorie free and adds that finishing sparkle.

Lemon juice is a marvelous flavor enhancer for many types of beverages (including, of course, lemonade, at only 107 calories a cup), so it's worth knowing how to maximize this resource. To get the most juice out of a lemon, allow it to come to room temperature or soak it in warm water before cutting into it. If you need only a very small amount of lemon juice, make a hole in one end of a lemon with a food pick. Squeeze out the juice you need, then stop up the hole with the food pick. Store the lemon in the refrigerator until the next time you need a few drops of lemon juice. A lemon will yield two to three tablespoons of juice. And you can grate about three teaspoons of zest from the skin of an average-size lemon.

Fruit juices do have calories, but they're wholesome and far preferable to the sugar-laden sodas and pops that really don't take care of a thirst and do add pounds. These juices are permissible on most diets and certainly are nutritious. You can make delicious punches by

The Calorie Count of Some Fruit Juices

Juice	Calories per Cup	Juice	Calories per Cup
Apple	116	Grapefruit	96
Apricot	122	Orange	112
Carrot	96	Papaya	120
Cranberry	147	Pineapple	140
Grape	156	Tangerine	108

combining several juices, or mixing them with soda water, herbal tea, or water.

Serve beverages that complement the desserts you make. Don't offer a tart drink with a sweet dessert. Grapefruit juice or combination grapefruit-orange juice would be a good choice with a lemon or lime pie. Apple juice is a perfect companion for a sweet cake.

In making diet drinks, replace milk or cream with skim milk. Yogurt is fine for occasional use as a drink ingredient. Homemade skim milk yogurt has fewer calories than the commercial low-fat yogurt.

Teas Are Easy and Offer Varied Choices

Herbal teas offer an opportunity to experiment with a variety of flavors. You can make them from either fresh or dried herbs. But since dried herbs are concentrated, you need to use only about half the amount you would when using fresh herbs. Although herbs differ in strength, when in doubt, figure one teaspoon of dried, or two teaspoons of fresh herbs for every cup of boiling water.

Herbs used to make teas come from the flowers, leaves, seeds, or bark of plants. Lemon verbena and lemon balm teas, my favorites, are delicious alone, hot or cold, or in combination with other herbs. The lovely lemon flavor enhances almost any other herb.

Because herbal teas have no calories, you can feel free to add a bit of sweetener if you wish. As an added bonus, soothing, even curative, properties are traditionally attributed to herbal teas.

Herbs to Use for Making Teas

A tea made from any of these herbs serves as a tasty distraction from high-calorie snacks.

Agrimony	Calamint	Dill	Marigold petals	Rue
Balm	Chamomile	Hyssop	Parsley	Sage
Bergamot	Costmary	Lemon verbena	Peppermint	Savory
Betony	Dandelion	Lovage	Rosemary	Sweet cicely

Cake Roll Pruneau

1 recipe for Jelly Roll Cake
   (page 54)
1 cup pitted prunes
2 cups water
¼ cup honey
½ teaspoon ground cinnamon
1 slice lemon
½ cup part-skim ricotta cheese

Bake Jelly Roll Cake according to directions.

In a medium-size saucepan, combine prunes, water, honey, cinnamon, and lemon. Bring to a boil. Reduce heat, cover, and simmer for 45 minutes.

Remove from heat and strain, reserving juice. Discard lemon. Set aside to cool. In a food processor, puree prunes. Add ricotta and process until smooth. If mixture is too thick to be spreadable, add reserved juice, a tablespoon at a time, until desired consistency is reached. Spread on cake and roll up. Cover and chill.

Slice to serve.

Makes 12 servings
(151 calories per serving)

Pineapple Charlotte

10 Ladyfingers (page 108)
 2 envelopes unflavored gelatin
½ cup water
1½ cups skim milk
½ cup honey
 3 eggs
1½ cups unsweetened pineapple
   juice
1 teaspoon orange extract

Spray bottom and sides of a 6-cup mold with vegetable spray. Line with Ladyfingers.

Sprinkle gelatin over water and set aside to soften for 5 minutes.

In a large saucepan, heat together skim milk and honey to scalding.

In a medium-size bowl, beat eggs for 1 minute. Whisk some of the hot milk mixture into eggs. Return to milk in pan and heat over medium heat, stirring constantly, until mixture starts to thicken. Stir in gelatin and continue cooking until it dissolves. Remove from heat and stir in juice and extract. Pour into a medium-size bowl and chill until thickened but not set. Beat until fluffy, turn into prepared mold, and chill until set.

Unmold onto a plate just before serving.

Makes 8 servings
(191 calories per serving)

Jelly Roll Cake

This recipe is the basis for the classic jelly roll cake.
Fill it with any of the filling recipes in the book.

5 eggs, separated
¼ teaspoon cream of tartar
3 tablespoons honey
1 teaspoon vanilla extract

½ cup sifted whole wheat
   flour
½ cup sifted unbleached
   white flour

Preheat oven to 350°F. Line a 15 × 10-inch baking pan with parchment paper.

In a medium-size bowl, beat egg whites until foamy. Sprinkle in cream of tartar and continue beating until stiff peaks form.

In a large bowl, beat egg yolks until light colored. Add honey and vanilla and beat for 7 minutes, or until very thick.

Sift together whole wheat flour and unbleached white flour into a small bowl, whisking to blend. Fold into beaten egg yolks. Fold in beaten whites and spread on prepared pan. Bake on middle shelf of oven for 12 minutes.

Sprinkle a tea towel lightly with flour. Turn cake out onto it. Carefully peel off parchment paper and roll cake and towel together, rolling from the short end of the cake. Allow to cool completely. Unroll and trim edges.

Makes 10 servings
(105 calories per serving)

Carob Thins

*This elegantly delicate cookie is one of
my favorites.*

    6 tablespoons butter, softened
    ¼ cup honey
    2 teaspoons vanilla extract
    1 cup whole wheat pastry flour
    1 cup unbleached white flour
    2 tablespoons carob powder
    ¼ teaspoon ground cinnamon
    2 tablespoons water

Preheat oven to 350°F. Line a 12 × 16-inch baking sheet (without sides) with foil (dull side up).

In a large bowl, cream together butter, honey, and vanilla.

Sift together whole wheat pastry flour, unbleached white flour, carob, and cinnamon into a medium-size bowl. Gradually mix into butter mixture, adding water as needed to form a stiff but workable dough. Shape dough into 2 rectangles. Place 1 piece of dough in center of prepared baking sheet. Top with piece of waxed paper the size of the baking sheet. Roll rectangle out to 11 × 14 inches on baking sheet. Remove waxed paper and cut dough into 36 squares. Bake on middle shelf of oven for 10 minutes.

Carefully remove to wire rack to cool. Repeat with other piece of dough on a cold baking sheet.

*Makes 6 dozen cookies
(25 calories per cookie)*

Luscious Citrus Pie

    4 Ladyfingers (page 108)
    1½ tablespoons unflavored gelatin
    1½ cups freshly squeezed orange
         juice, strained
    ⅓ cup honey
    2 egg yolks, at room temperature
    3 egg whites, at room temperature
    ⅛ teaspoon cream of tartar
    1 teaspoon vanilla extract

Lightly spray a 9-inch pie plate with vegetable spray.

Split Ladyfingers lengthwise. Then cut each piece in half crosswise. Stand pieces around edge of pie plate, scallop side up.

In the top of a double boiler, sprinkle gelatin over orange juice. Set aside to soften for 5 minutes.

In a small bowl, beat honey and egg yolks together until thickened. Whisk into softened gelatin mixture, set over simmering water, and heat for 8 minutes, stirring constantly. Turn into a large bowl and refrigerate until thickened but not set, stirring frequently. (Mixture takes about 45 minutes to thicken.)

In a medium-size bowl, beat egg whites until foamy. Add cream of tartar and vanilla and continue beating until stiff peaks form. Fold into orange mixture and turn into prepared pie plate, smoothing top. Chill until set.

*Makes 8 servings
(107 calories per serving)*

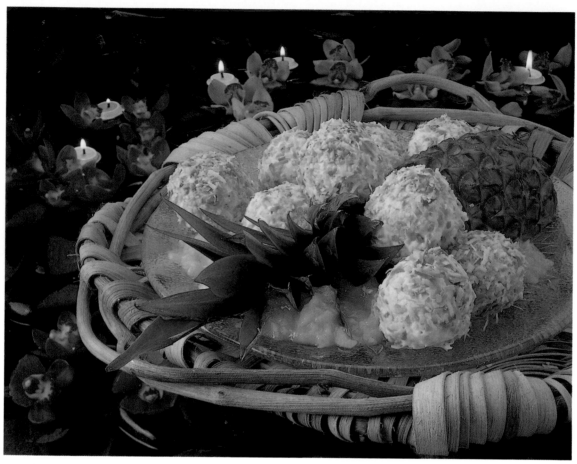

Hawaiian Snow Balls (page 60)

Banana Cream Pie

1 recipe for Meringue Pie Shell
   (page 117)
2 ripe bananas
3 cups Slim Pastry Cream
   (page 270)
¼ cup unsweetened flaked coconut

Bake pie shell according to directions. Allow to cool.

Thinly slice bananas. In a medium-size bowl, mix them with pastry cream. Turn into pie shell. Sprinkle with coconut and serve at once.

Makes 10 servings
(128 calories per serving)

Light Carrot Cake

⅓ cup whole wheat pastry flour
⅓ cup unbleached white flour
2 tablespoons cornstarch
1 teaspoon baking powder
½ teaspoon ground ginger
½ teaspoon ground nutmeg
3 eggs, separated
¼ teaspoon cream of tartar
⅓ cup honey
1 teaspoon vanilla extract
1 cup grated cooked carrots

Preheat oven to 350°F. Spray a 10-inch tube pan with vegetable spray.

Sift together whole wheat pastry flour, unbleached white flour, cornstarch, baking powder, ginger, and nutmeg into a small bowl. Whisk to blend well.

In a medium-size bowl, beat egg whites until foamy. Add cream of tartar and continue beating until stiff peaks form.

In a large bowl, beat together egg yolks, honey, and vanilla until light colored and thick, about 7 minutes. Fold in dry ingredients. Fold in carrots, then beaten egg whites.

Turn into prepared pan and bake on middle shelf of oven until top springs back when lightly pressed, 20 to 25 minutes.

Invert pan on wire rack and cool completely before removing cake from pan.

Makes 10 servings
(100 calories per serving)

Carob Chippers

½ cup whole wheat pastry flour
½ cup unbleached white flour
2 teaspoons baking powder
¼ cup butter, softened
¼ cup honey
2 tablespoons maple syrup
1 tablespoon vanilla extract
⅓ cup carob chips

Preheat oven to 350°F. Spray 2 baking sheets with vegetable spray.

In a small bowl, whisk whole wheat pastry flour, unbleached white flour, and baking powder together to blend.

In a medium-size bowl, beat together butter and honey until fluffy. Beat in maple syrup and vanilla. Gradually beat in dry ingredients. Fold in carob chips. Drop dough by teaspoonfuls onto 1 prepared baking sheet. Bake on middle shelf of oven until lightly browned, 8 to 10 minutes.

While cookies are baking, drop remaining dough onto second prepared baking sheet. Put in oven when first batch is cooked. Remove cookies from baking sheets and cool on wire racks.

Makes 3 dozen cookies
(41 calories per cookie)

Individual Strawberry Cheese Puddings

1 16-ounce package unsweetened frozen strawberries, thawed
1 envelope unflavored gelatin
1 cup part-skim ricotta cheese
¼ cup honey
¾ cup evaporated skim milk, chilled
¾ cup Perfect Pineapple Sauce (page 60), divided

Drain strawberries well, reserving both juice and berries. Pour juice into a small saucepan. Sprinkle gelatin over juice and set aside for 5 minutes to soften. Heat over medium heat, stirring constantly, until gelatin dissolves. Remove from heat and set aside to cool.

In a medium-size bowl, beat ricotta and honey together until fluffy. Beat in cooled gelatin and chill until thickened but not set, about 30 minutes, stirring occasionally, so edges won't set.

In a medium-size bowl, beat evaporated skim milk until fluffy. Fold into gelatin mixture along with strawberries. Divide among 6 small dessert dishes and chill until set.

To serve, unmold and top each pudding with 2 tablespoons of the pineapple sauce.

Makes 6 servings
(118 calories per serving)

Raisin Pear Bread Pudding

4 slices whole grain bread
3 eggs, separated
⅛ teaspoon cream of tartar
2 tablespoons honey
1¾ cups skim milk
1 teaspoon vanilla extract
½ teaspoon ground cinnamon
1 large fresh pear, peeled, cored, and chopped
¼ cup raisins, plumped

Preheat oven to 350°F. Spray a 2-quart casserole with vegetable spray.

Break bread into chunks.

In a medium-size bowl, beat egg whites until foamy. Add cream of tartar and continue beating until stiff peaks form.

In a large bowl, beat together egg yolks and honey briefly. Mix in skim milk, vanilla, and cinnamon, beating just to mix. Add bread, stirring until saturated.

Mix pears and raisins into bread mixture. Fold in beaten egg whites and turn into prepared casserole. Bake on middle shelf of oven for about 1 hour. Serve warm or cold.

Makes 8 servings
(125 calories per serving)

Spicy Pears

A lovely juicy pear dessert.

2 tablespoons honey
1 tablespoon butter
1 teaspoon ground cinnamon
¼ teaspoon ground ginger
1 cup cornflakes
4 large fresh Bartlett pears
2 tablespoons apple juice

Preheat oven to 350°F.

In a small saucepan, heat together honey, butter, cinnamon, and ginger until butter is melted. Mix with cornflakes.

Peel, core, and thinly slice pears into a 9-inch pie plate. Pour apple juice over pear slices. Distribute cornflake mixture evenly over top and bake on middle shelf of oven until pears are tender, about 20 minutes. Serve warm or cold.

Makes 6 servings
(141 calories per serving)

Reduced Calorie Peanut Butter

The use of dry roasted peanuts is what reduces the calories in this diet version of one of America's favorite foods.

2 cups dry roasted peanuts

In a food processor, process nuts until they are the consistency of paste, adding water by tablespoonfuls to make it spreadable. Stop machine occasionally and scrape down sides of bowl and release nuts trapped under blade. Store in refrigerator.

Makes about 1½ cups
(70 calories per tablespoon)

Perfect Pineapple Sauce

1 tablespoon cornstarch
¼ cup freshly squeezed
     orange juice

2 tablespoons honey
1 20-ounce can unsweet-
     ened crushed pineapple

Stir cornstarch into orange juice in a small saucepan. Add honey, blending well. Add pineapple and cook over medium heat, stirring constantly, until sauce thickens.

Makes about 2 cups
(15 calories per tablespoon)

Hawaiian Snow Balls

2 cups Vanilla Ice Milk (page 79)
½ cup unsweetened flaked coconut
½ cup Perfect Pineapple Sauce
     (page 60)

Line a small baking sheet with waxed paper. Make 4 perfectly rounded, ½-cup scoops of vanilla ice milk. Place them on prepared baking sheet and freeze until very firm.

Preheat oven to 350°F. Put coconut in shallow pan, and toast on middle shelf of oven, stirring occasionally, until lightly browned, about 10 minutes. Cool slightly, then roll ice milk balls in toasted coconut. Return to freezer for at least 30 minutes.

Serve with 2 tablespoons of pineapple sauce on each ball.

Makes 4 servings
(179 calories per serving)

Peanut Butter Apples

A wholesome, easy dessert, quick and satisfying.

1 apple
4 teaspoons Reduced Calorie
     Peanut Butter (page 59),
     divided
2 teaspoons Coconut Sugar
     (page 66), divided

Core, but do not peel, apple; then cut it into quarters.

Spread 1 teaspoon of the peanut butter on cut sides of each quarter. Sprinkle each piece with ½ teaspoon of the Coconut Sugar.

Makes 4 servings
(48 calories per serving)

Ring of Plenty

1 recipe for **Fresh Orange Gelatin**
  (page 248)
1 apple
1 fresh pear
2 tablespoons freshly squeezed
  lemon juice
1 seedless orange
16 unsweetened frozen cherries,
  thawed

Make gelatin according to directions up to the point when it is thickened but not set. Then beat gelatin until foamy. Pour into a lightly oiled 4- or 6-cup ring mold. Chill until set.

Core and slice, but do not peel, apple and pear. Toss with lemon juice in a medium-size bowl. Peel and section orange, removing pith. Toss all fruit together.

Unmold orange ring on platter and fill with fruit. Serve at once.

Makes 8 servings
(64 calories per serving)

Luscious Lemon Cheesecake

A special dessert for a special day.

2 envelopes unflavored gelatin
1 cup freshly squeezed lemon
  juice
16 ounces low-fat cottage cheese
2 tablespoons butter, softened
¾ cup plus 1 tablespoon honey,
  divided
4 eggs, separated
⅛ teaspoon cream of tartar
¼ cup **Light Lemon Cookie** crumbs
  (page 133)

Spray bottom and sides of a 9-inch springform pan with vegetable spray.

In the top of a double boiler, sprinkle gelatin over lemon juice. Set aside for 5 minutes to soften.

In a blender or food processor, beat together cottage cheese and butter.

Stir ¾ cup of the honey into gelatin mixture. Beat egg yolks slightly and add to gelatin. Heat over hot water, stirring constantly, for 10 minutes. Slowly beat hot mixture into cheese mixture. Chill until thickened but not set, stirring frequently.

In a medium-size bowl, beat egg whites until foamy. Add cream of tartar and continue beating, drizzling in remaining honey, until stiff but not dry. Stir a little egg white into gelatin mixture to lighten. Fold in remaining egg whites and turn into prepared pan. Sprinkle with cookie crumbs and chill until set.

To serve, run knife around edge of cheesecake and release springform.

Makes 12 to 16 servings
(164 to 122 calories per serving)

Squash Custard

2 eggs, separated
⅛ teaspoon cream of tartar
2 tablespoons honey
1 cup cooked pureed winter
   squash
¾ cup skim milk
1 teaspoon ground cinnamon
¼ teaspoon ground nutmeg
¼ teaspoon ground ginger

Preheat oven to 325°F. Spray a 1-quart casserole with vegetable spray.

In a medium-size bowl, beat egg whites until foamy. Add cream of tartar and continue beating until stiff peaks form.

In a large bowl, beat egg yolks and honey. Add remaining ingredients and beat just to mix. Fold in beaten egg whites and turn into prepared casserole. Bake on middle shelf of oven until a cake tester inserted into center comes out clean, about 45 minutes. Serve warm or cold.

Makes 6 servings
(75 calories per serving)

Almond Coconut Chiffon Pie

1 recipe for Skinny Piecrust
   (page 6)
1 cup skim milk
3 eggs, separated
3 tablespoons honey
1 envelope unflavored gelatin
1 teaspoon almond extract
⅛ teaspoon cream of tartar
½ cup unsweetened flaked coconut

Line a 10-inch pie plate just to the rim with pastry, and bake according to directions. Set aside to cool.

In a medium-size bowl, beat together skim milk, egg yolks, and honey. Pour into a medium-size saucepan. Sprinkle gelatin over top and heat over medium heat, stirring constantly, for 5 minutes. Stir in almond extract. Turn into a large bowl and chill until thickened but not set, about 1½ hours, stirring every 30 minutes.

In a medium-size bowl, beat egg whites and cream of tartar until stiff peaks form. Fold egg whites into gelatin mixture. Fold in coconut and turn into prepared piecrust. Chill until ready to serve.

Makes 10 servings
(110 calories per serving)

Luscious Lemon Cheesecake (page 61)

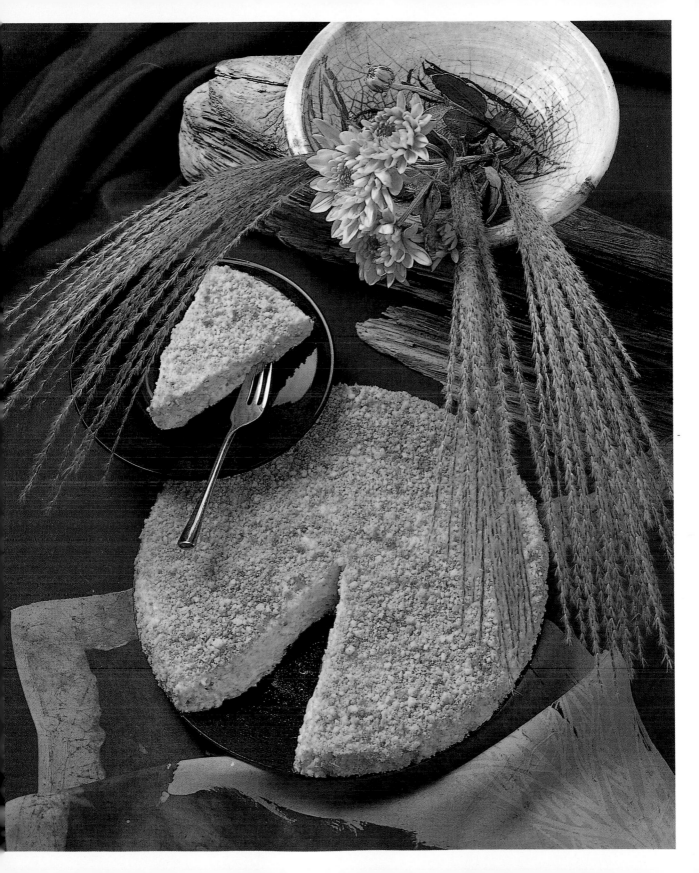

★ Orange Meringue Cups

3 large seedless oranges
2 egg whites
⅛ teaspoon cream of tartar
3 tablespoons unsweetened flaked
   coconut
6 seedless green or red grapes,
   divided

Preheat oven to 350°F.

Cut oranges into halves. With a serrated knife, cut between skins and pulp. Run knife between pulp and membranes, loosening sections. Place orange halves in a muffin tin, pulp side up.

In a medium-size bowl, beat egg whites until foamy. Add cream of tartar and continue beating until stiff peaks form. Fold in coconut and pile mixture on orange halves. Bake on bottom shelf of oven until meringue browns, about 10 minutes.

Cool and top each with a grape.

Makes 6 servings
(42 calories per serving)

Saint Paddy's Day Mint Treat

This is a delightfully refreshing dessert that makes a beautiful presentation.

2 envelopes unflavored gelatin
1½ cups skim milk
2 egg yolks
¼ cup honey
1 tablespoon vanilla extract
1½ teaspoons peppermint extract
3 drops natural green food
   coloring, optional

4 egg whites
⅛ teaspoon cream of tartar
⅔ cup instant nonfat dry milk
⅔ cup ice water
1 cup Creamy Carob Sauce
   (page 205)

In a small saucepan, sprinkle gelatin over skim milk. Set aside for 5 minutes to soften.

In a small bowl, whisk egg yolks until thick and yellow.

Add honey to milk mixture and heat over medium heat, stirring until mixture is scalding (150°F on a candy thermometer). Remove from heat and whisk a little hot milk into beaten yolks. Return yolk mixture to saucepan, whisking constantly. Cook over low heat, stirring constantly, until mixture reaches 175°F on a candy thermometer. Turn into a large bowl, and mix in extracts and food coloring, if desired.

In a medium-size bowl, beat egg whites until foamy. Add cream of tartar and continue beating until stiff peaks form.

In a large bowl, beat together instant nonfat dry milk and ice water until soft peaks form.

Fold instant nonfat dry milk into egg mixture, then fold in egg whites. Rinse a 6-cup mold with cold water. Turn mixture into it, smoothing top. Refrigerate until set.

To unmold, dip mold briefly in hot water. Place serving dish on top of mold and invert. Serve with Creamy Carob Sauce.

Makes 8 servings
(190 calories per serving)

Stuffed Baked Pears

These pears are equally delicious warm or chilled.

¾ cup water, divided
½ cup grape juice
½ teaspoon ground cinnamon
⅛ teaspoon ground cloves
4 fresh pears
2 tablespoons raisins
2 tablespoons chopped walnuts
1 tablespoon cornstarch

Preheat oven to 350°F.

In a small saucepan, bring ½ cup of the water, grape juice, cinnamon, and cloves to a boil. Reduce heat and cook for 1 minute. Remove from heat.

Cut tops, about 1 inch down, off pears and reserve. Peel and core pears, leaving bottoms intact.

In a small bowl, mix together raisins and walnuts and stuff pears with them. Replace tops. Stand pears up in a casserole. Pour grape sauce over them. Cover and bake until fruit is soft, about 1 hour.

Pour sauce from casserole into a small saucepan. In a jar with a tight-fitting lid, shake together the remaining water and cornstarch. Stir into sauce and heat, stirring constantly, until thickened. Pour over pears and set aside to cool.

Makes 4 servings
(167 calories per serving)

Frozen Pudding

2 egg whites
⅛ teaspoon cream of tartar
2 cups Very Vanilla Pudding
    (page 84), cooled slightly but
    not set
1 banana
¼ cup raisins, plumped
8 seedless red grapes

Line 8 cups of a muffin tin with paper liners.

In a medium-size bowl, beat egg whites until foamy. Add cream of tartar and continue beating until stiff peaks form. Fold into cooled pudding.

Chop banana. Fold along with raisins into pudding. Divide among paper liners and freeze.

When frozen, remove pudding-filled liners from tin and store in a plastic bag in freezer.

To serve, decorate each serving with a grape.

Makes 8 servings
(95 calories per serving)

Coconut Sugar

This easy decoration can be used to dust cakes, candies, or fruits.

1¼ cups unsweetened flaked coconut

In a food processor, process coconut until it is the consistency of powdered sugar.

Makes 1 cup
(20 calories per tablespoon)

Super Spice Cake

You can add zip to a recipe with spices, and the number of calories you add is almost negligible.

- ½ **cup sifted whole wheat pastry flour**
- ½ **cup sifted unbleached white flour**
- 2 **teaspoons baking powder**
- 2 **teaspoons ground cinnamon**
- 1 **teaspoon ground nutmeg**
- 1 **teaspoon ground ginger**
- 5 **egg whites**
- ¼ **teaspoon cream of tartar**
- 3 **egg yolks**
- 1 **tablespoon vegetable oil**
- 1 **teaspoon vanilla extract**
- ½ **teaspoon orange extract**
- ¼ **cup honey**
- 1 **tablespoon molasses**

Preheat oven to 350°F.

Sift together whole wheat pastry flour, unbleached white flour, baking powder, cinnamon, nutmeg, and ginger into a medium-size bowl. Stir with wire whisk to blend well.

In a large bowl, beat egg whites until foamy. Add cream of tartar and continue beating until stiff peaks form.

In a small bowl, beat together egg yolks, oil, extracts, honey, and molasses with same beaters. Add to dry ingredients, mixing well. Add a small amount of egg whites, stirring to lighten. Fold in remaining whites and turn into an 8 × 8-inch pan with a nonstick surface. Reduce heat to 325°F. Bake on middle shelf of oven for 40 to 45 minutes, or until a cake tester inserted near center comes out clean. Cool before serving.

Makes 12 servings
(98 calories per serving)

Rum-Tum-Diddle Soufflés

This easy, light-as-air dessert should be served warm.

3 egg whites
¼ teaspoon cream of tartar
3 tablespoons honey, divided
1 teaspoon vanilla extract
½ cup evaporated skim milk, chilled
½ teaspoon rum extract
8 tablespoons Ruby Raspberry Sauce (page 139), divided

Preheat oven to 350°F. Spray 8 8-ounce ovenproof custard cups or dishes with vegetable spray.

In a medium-size bowl, beat egg whites until foamy. Add cream of tartar, 2 tablespoons of the honey, and vanilla and continue beating until stiff peaks form.

In a large bowl, beat evaporated skim milk until foamy. Add remaining honey and rum extract and continue beating until soft peaks form. Fold beaten egg whites into beaten milk mixture. Turn into prepared custard cups or dishes and bake on bottom shelf of oven until soufflés have risen and are lightly browned.

Serve hot with a tablespoon of the Ruby Raspberry Sauce on each soufflé.

Makes 8 servings
(49 calories per serving)

Brandy Zabaglione

This dessert must be served as soon as it's made as it tends to separate on standing.

4 eggs, separated
2 tablespoons honey
1 teaspoon brandy extract
¼ teaspoon cream of tartar
1 teaspoon red currant jelly, divided

In the top of a double boiler set over simmering water, beat together egg yolks, honey, and brandy extract until mixture is thick and light colored, about 7 minutes.

In a medium-size bowl, beat egg whites until foamy. Sprinkle in cream of tartar and continue beating until stiff peaks form. Fold egg yolk mixture into beaten egg whites. Divide among 4 dessert glasses. Top each with ¼ teaspoon of the jelly and serve immediately.

Makes 4 servings
(118 calories per serving)

Tangy Tangerine Crepes

½ cup part-skim ricotta cheese
1 tablespoon skim milk
¼ teaspoon almond extract
8 Delicious Diet Crepes (page 33)
¼ cup butter
2 tablespoons honey
1 tablespoon cornstarch
1 cup freshly squeezed orange
   juice
1 tangerine, peeled, sectioned and
   pith removed

In a medium-size bowl, beat together ricotta, skim milk, and almond extract until fluffy. Divide among 8 crepes and spread the mixture down the center of each. Fold 1 side over filling, then the other side.

In a large skillet, melt butter. Stir in honey.

Dissolve cornstarch in orange juice. Add to skillet and stir constantly until thickened. Carefully place crepes in hot sauce. Cover, and heat for 5 minutes. Remove from heat. Decorate with tangerine sections and serve immediately.

Makes 8 servings
(146 calories per serving)

Lemon Sorbet

1 cup freshly squeezed lemon
   juice
3 cups water, divided
⅔ cup honey
1 teaspoon lemon extract
   natural yellow food coloring,
   optional

Strain lemon juice into a large bowl. Mix in 2½ cups of the water.

In a small saucepan, heat remaining water and honey until honey dissolves. Add to lemon juice in bowl. Mix in lemon extract and a few drops of food coloring, if desired.

Process mixture in an ice cream maker according to manufacturer's instructions, or turn mixture into a large pan and place in freezer until mushy but not solid. Remove from freezer, beat to break down ice crystals, and then return to freezer. Repeat this procedure twice. Freeze until ready to serve.

Makes about 10 servings
(58 calories per serving)

Almond Coconut Chiffon Pie (page 62)

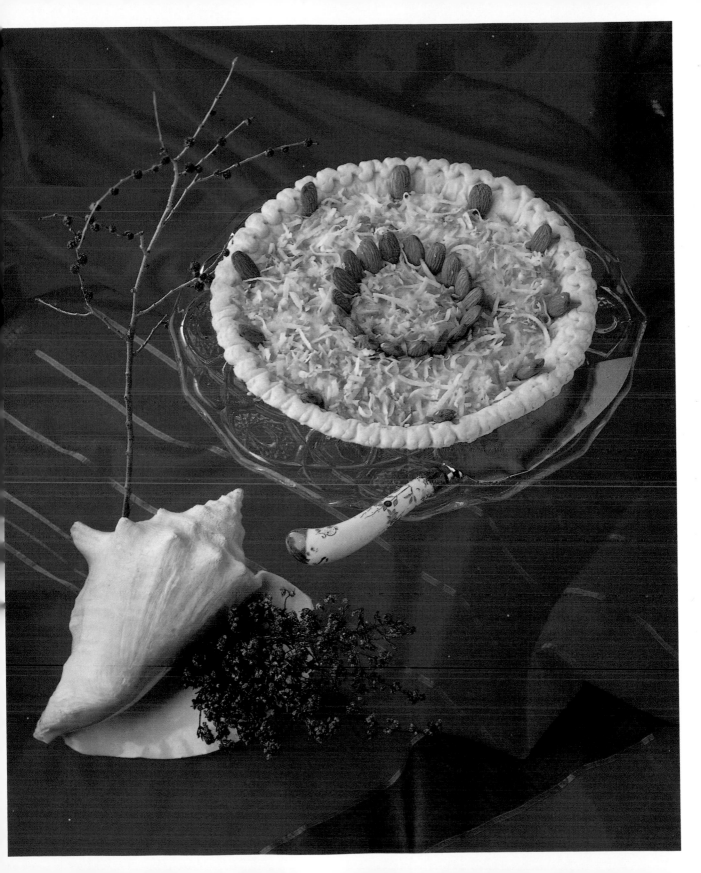

Tangerine Bread Pudding with Peach Sauce

Be sure to remove all the pith from the tangerine or the pudding will be bitter.

      3 eggs, separated, at room
        temperature
    ⅛ teaspoon cream of tartar
      2 tablespoons honey
  1⅔ cups evaporated skim milk
      1 teaspoon vanilla extract
    ½ teaspoon almond extract
    ½ teaspoon ground cinnamon
      4 slices whole wheat bread (with
        crusts), broken into chunks
      1 tangerine
    ½ cup Peach Sauce (page 132),
        divided

Preheat oven to 350°F. Spray a 2-quart casserole with vegetable spray.

In a medium-size bowl, beat egg whites until foamy. Add cream of tartar and continue beating until stiff peaks form.

In a large bowl, beat together egg yolks and honey just to blend. Mix in evaporated skim milk, extracts, and cinnamon, beating briefly. Add bread, stirring until it is saturated.

Peel tangerine and separate into sections, removing pith. Cut each section into fourths, removing seeds. Stir into bread mixture. Fold in beaten egg whites and turn into prepared casserole. Bake on middle shelf of oven for 45 minutes.

Serve warm or cold. Top each serving with 1 tablespoon of the Peach Sauce.

Makes 8 servings
(134 calories per serving)

Orange Date Cookies

    ½ cup whole wheat flour
    ½ cup unbleached white flour
      1 teaspoon baking powder
    ¼ cup butter, cut into pieces
    ⅓ cup unsweetened flaked coconut
    ½ cup freshly squeezed orange
        juice
      2 tablespoons honey
      1 teaspoon vanilla extract
      1 teaspoon orange extract
      1 egg, beaten
      9 dates, quartered

Preheat oven to 350°F. Spray 2 baking sheets with vegetable spray.

In a medium-size bowl, mix together whole wheat flour, unbleached white flour, and baking powder with a whisk. Cut butter into flour mixture with pastry blender until mixture resembles crumbs. Mix in coconut.

In a small bowl, combine orange juice, honey, and extracts. Thoroughly stir into flour mixture. Mix in egg. Drop batter by teaspoonfuls onto prepared baking sheets. Put a piece of date on top of each portion of batter. Bake each batch on middle shelf of oven for 10 minutes.

Cool on wire rack.

Makes 3 dozen cookies
(40 calories per cookie)

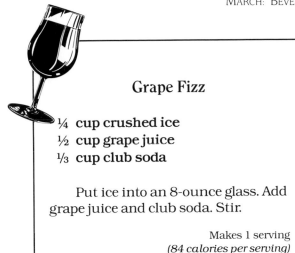

Grape Fizz

¼ cup crushed ice
½ cup grape juice
⅓ cup club soda

Put ice into an 8-ounce glass. Add grape juice and club soda. Stir.

Makes 1 serving
(84 calories per serving)

Baked Jungle Treat

2 ripe bananas
2 teaspoons butter, melted
¼ cup Coconut Sugar (page 66)

Preheat oven to 400°F. Spray a baking sheet with vegetable spray.

Cut bananas into halves, lengthwise. Brush all surfaces with melted butter and roll bananas in Coconut Sugar. Place, cut side down, on prepared baking sheet and bake on middle shelf of oven until lightly browned, 5 to 7 minutes. Serve immediately.

Makes 4 servings
(78 calories per serving)

Carob Chip Pie

1 recipe for Meringue Pie Shell
    (page 117)
2 cups Carob Chip Pudding
    (page 201)
4 whole fresh strawberries,
    optional

Bake pie shell according to directions. Cool.

Fill meringue shell with thoroughly cooled Carob Chip Pudding.

Cut strawberries into halves lengthwise and decorate pie, if desired. Chill until serving time.

Makes 8 servings
(92 calories per serving)

Nice Spice Popcorn

A handy sweet you can carry away from the table as a low-cal nibble for a later time.

2 tablespoons butter
1 tablespoon honey
1 teaspoon ground cinnamon
¼ teaspoon ground nutmeg
¼ teaspoon ground ginger
8 cups hot popcorn

In a small saucepan, melt butter and honey. Add spices and stir until dissolved. Toss with popcorn and serve immediately, 1 cup per person.

Makes 8 servings
(48 calories per serving)

APRIL

Diet and Exercise

				April Fools' Day 1	2	3
FRUIT OF THE MONTH: **STRAWBERRIES** *DESSERT OF THE MONTH:* **GOOD OLD STRAWBERRY SHORTCAKE** *DRINK OF THE MONTH:* **STRAWBERRY FIZZ**				PEAR SURPRISE	STRAWBERRY BANANA CREAM	COFFEE BAVARIAN CREAM
4 ORANGE PINEAPPLE SHERBET	5 OLD-FASHIONED CUSTARD	6 CAROB CONFECTIONS	7 GOOD OLD STRAWBERRY SHORTCAKE ★	8 BANANA MINT TREATS	9 VANILLA ICE MILK	10 FLUFFY ALMOND TAPIOCA
11 PEANUT BUTTER DROP COOKIES	12 STRAWBERRY GRAPE PIE	13 PEACH SOUFFLÉ	14 APRICOT BRANDY ICE	*Easter* 15 HAPPY EASTER BASKETS	16 CAROB CRUMB APPLES	17 VERY VANILLA PUDDING
18 PIÑA COLADA PIE	19 STRAWBERRY BREAD PUDDING	20 ALMOND YOGURT	21 APPLESAUCE FLUFF	22 YOGURT-TOPPED GINGERBREAD	23 COOL STRAWBERRY SOUP	24 SENSATIONAL FRUIT PIE
25 FROZEN BANANAS	26 MELLOW MERINGUES	27 ½ CUP SLICED STRAWBERRIES	28 PINEAPPLE FROMAGE	29 MANGO STRAWBERRY CREPE STACKS	30 COTTAGE CHEESE PIE	

72

Happy Easter Baskets (page 83)

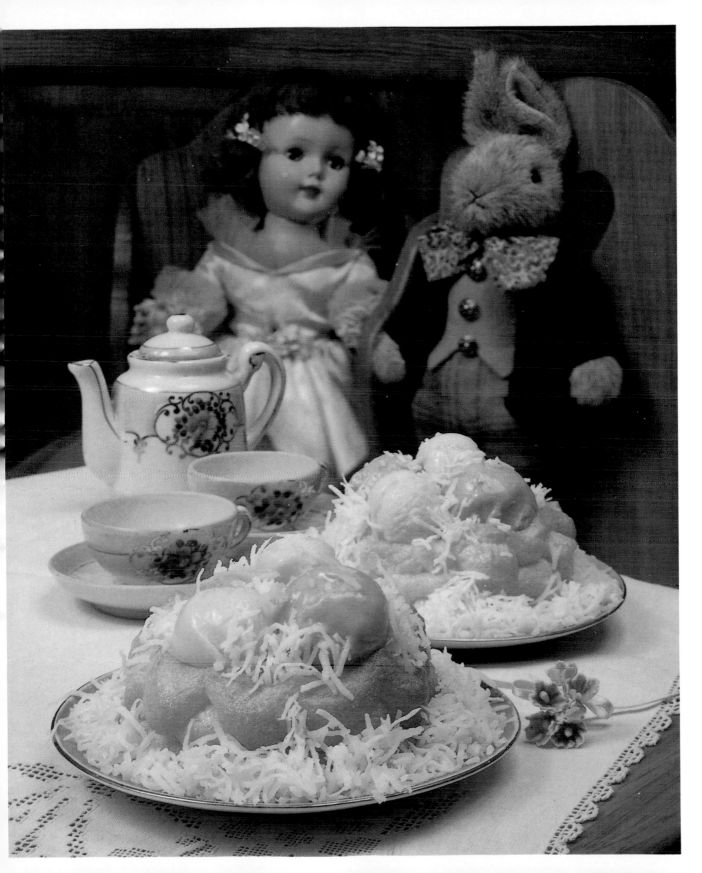

If you weren't interested in being slender and healthy, you probably wouldn't be reading this book. Eating correctly is certainly a large part of total fitness, but it is only part. Firming up completes the picture. Although you need exercise year round, I've selected April as exercise month. With summer on the horizon and the winter blahs but a memory, it's an excellent time to begin an exercise program. After all, the time for bathing suits and other light clothes that don't always cover trouble spots is right around the corner.

Do get your doctor's permission before embarking on any exercise program. But whether you're eight or eighty-eight, there are many benefits to be derived from physical activity, and whatever your age or physical condition there's some kind of exercise that's right for you. Even a program of moderate exercise, done on a regular basis, will burn up small amounts of calories and help with weight control.

When you're firming up, the idea is to stretch your muscles just a little beyond what they're accustomed to. Your muscle tone will increase as you continue to exercise over the weeks and months. Since I've started doing specific exercises three times a week and walking daily, I not only feel better physically, but my outlook on life is wonderful. And I sleep better, too. This isn't just coincidence. Exercise relieves stress by causing certain chemical changes in the body. After exercising you should feel full of energy and "high" on life.

Many people avoid exercise in the mistaken belief that it increases appetite. The truth is that it decreases your desire for food. You're burning off fat, and so that fat no longer needs calories on which to run.

Always warm up before you do any strenuous exercise. Your muscles need to stretch gently before a workout. Failure to take this simple step has resulted in many a strained or torn ligament. It's also vital to the cardiovascular system to warm down after exercise.

The proper attire may put you in an exercise mood. Select an outfit that's loose fitting, comfortable, and absorbent . . . one that will bend and stretch easily with your body.

Music makes exercising seem easier, keeping motion constant and rhythmic. It's more fun to move to a beat. If you're not used to exercise, start with a slow, steady tune. You'll be surprised at how soon you're ready for a fast-paced piece. Television offers several lively exercise programs. They make it almost like having a friend right there to exercise with you.

An exercise session should be uninterrupted, not only for the sake of convenience, but also so you won't lose the benefits of your warm-ups. Take the phone off the hook, or tell your family and friends not to call you during your exercise time.

Exercise at your own pace. It's all right to start slowly and build up to whatever you're comfortable doing. You should feel your muscles working, but real pain or very hard, rapid breathing are indications you're overdoing it.

I've often heard that for every inch taller you sit, you look five pounds thinner. So include an exercise to strengthen your back and improve your posture in your program.

Walking is a gold star exercise that almost anyone can do. You won't lose a great deal of weight this way, but it's a fantastic way to maintain weight loss if you do it correctly. Hold in your stomach, stand tall, and walk briskly with your arms swinging. Start with a half mile and work up. You can add a half mile to your walking program every week or so until you build it up to a distance that's comfortable for you and fits into your time schedule.

There's no medical evidence to back up the idea that you shouldn't walk after eating, providing you're in good health and not suffering from a coronary insufficiency.

Walking offers many benefits other than maintaining weight. It strengthens the heart, tightens the stomach muscles, and reduces tension. And walking seems to be something most people can stick to. There are fewer drop-outs than in other more strenuous exercise programs. There are also very few injuries.

Coffee Bavarian Cream

1¼ cups skim milk
 2 eggs, separated
 2 envelopes unflavored gelatin
 ⅓ cup honey, divided
 1 tablespoon decaffeinated
    instant coffee
1½ teaspoons vanilla extract
 ⅛ teaspoon cream of tartar
 1 cup evaporated skim milk,
    chilled
12 mandarin orange sections,
    optional

In the top of a double boiler, beat together skim milk and egg yolks. Sprinkle gelatin over mixture and set aside for 5 minutes to soften. Add 2 tablespoons of the honey and coffee, set over hot, not boiling, water and cook, stirring constantly, until gelatin is dissolved. Remove from heat and mix in vanilla. Chill until thickened but not set, no longer than 30 minutes. Whisk briefly until smooth.

In a medium-size bowl, beat egg whites until foamy. Add cream of tartar and drizzle in remaining honey. Continue to beat until stiff peaks form. Fold egg whites into gelatin mixture.

In a chilled, medium-size bowl, beat evaporated skim milk to the consistency of whipped cream. Fold into gelatin mixture. Turn into a wet 8-cup mold and chill until set.

Unmold and decorate with orange sections, if desired.

Makes 12 servings
(76 calories per serving)

Pear Surprise

 2 cups water
 3 fresh pears
 ⅓ cup Light Lemon Cookie crumbs
    (page 133)
 1 4 ½-ounce jar strained plums
 ¼ teaspoon rum extract
 1 tablespoon butter

In a large saucepan, bring water to a boil. Add pears, reduce heat, and poach for 10 minutes. Remove with a slotted spoon and set aside to cool.

Preheat oven to 350°F. Spray a 9-inch pie plate with vegetable spray.

In a small bowl, mix together cookie crumbs, plums, and rum extract.

In a small saucepan, melt butter.

When pears are cool enough to handle, peel, halve, and core them. Place, hollow side up, in prepared pie plate. Fill each indentation with crumb mixture. Lightly brush pears and filling with melted butter. Place on middle shelf of oven and bake until fruit is soft, about 10 minutes.

Makes 6 servings
(150 calories per serving)

Orange Pineapple Sherbet

1 envelope unflavored gelatin
½ cup water
⅓ cup honey
1 6-ounce can unsweetened
    frozen orange juice
    concentrate
1 6-ounce can unsweetened
    frozen pineapple juice
    concentrate
1½ cups skim milk
1 cup buttermilk

In a small saucepan, sprinkle gelatin over water. Set aside for 5 minutes to soften. Place over low heat. Add honey and stir until gelatin is dissolved.

In a large bowl, mix together juice concentrates, skim milk, and buttermilk. Stir in gelatin mixture.

Process mixture in an ice cream maker according to manufacturer's instructions, or turn mixture into a large pan and place in freezer until thickened but not solid. Remove from freezer, beat to break down ice crystals, and then return to freezer. Repeat this procedure twice, turning mixture into 2 1-quart containers the last time. Freeze until ready to serve.

Makes 8 servings
(184 calories per serving)

Cool Strawberry Soup

This cooling summer dessert is so delicious, I sometimes make it my entire lunch.

3 cups unsweetened frozen straw-
    berries, thawed
⅓ cup white grape juice
½ cup freshly squeezed orange
    juice
1 tablespoon cornstarch
2 tablespoons honey
¼ teaspoon ground cinnamon
1 teaspoon vanilla extract
1 cup plain low-fat yogurt

In a food processor, puree strawberries. Turn into a medium-size saucepan.

In a jar with a tight-fitting lid, shake together grape juice, orange juice, and cornstarch. Add to strawberries. Stir in honey and cinnamon, and cook over medium heat, stirring constantly, until thickened, 5 to 10 minutes. Remove from heat and mix in vanilla. Cool, then whisk in yogurt just until blended. Chill before serving.

Makes 6 servings
(94 calories per serving)

Banana Mint Treats

½ teaspoon peppermint extract
¼ cup Creamy Carob Sauce
   (page 205), divided
2 cups Vanilla Ice Milk (page 79),
   divided
1 ripe banana

In a small bowl, mix peppermint extract into carob sauce.

Put ¼ cup Vanilla Ice Milk into each of 4 dessert dishes. Slice 2 banana rounds into each dessert dish. Top with ¼ cup of the Vanilla Ice Milk. Repeat banana layer and top each serving with 1 tablespoon of the carob sauce. Serve immediately.

Makes 4 servings
(187 calories per serving)

Yogurt-Topped Gingerbread

1 cup plain nonfat yogurt
2 tablespoons freshly squeezed
   lemon juice
1 tablespoon honey
1 banana
   Gingerbread Squares, uncut
   (page 202)

In a small bowl, mix together yogurt, lemon juice, and honey. Chop banana and add to yogurt. Spread mixture on top of Gingerbread. Cut into 9 pieces and serve immediately.

Makes 9 servings
(152 calories per serving)

Strawberry Banana Cream

2 cups skim milk, divided
⅔ cup nonfat dry milk
2 medium-size ripe bananas
1 teaspoon freshly squeezed
   lemon juice
2 tablespoons cornstarch
1½ tablespoons honey
1½ teaspoons vanilla extract
1 cup sliced fresh strawberries

In the top of a double boiler, whisk together 1½ cups of the skim milk and nonfat dry milk.

In a small bowl, thoroughly mash together bananas and lemon juice, whisking briskly to blend. Whisk bananas into milk in top of double boiler. Shake together remaining skim milk and cornstarch in a tightly covered jar. Whisk into milk-banana mixture, set over boiling water, and cook, stirring constantly, until mixture thickens, about 8 minutes. Remove from heat and stir in honey and vanilla. Mix in strawberries and chill well before serving.

Makes 8 to 10 servings
(86 to 68 calories per serving)

Skinny Shortcakes

These are wonderful for making fruit shortcakes.

½ cup whole wheat pastry
   flour
½ cup unbleached white flour
1 teaspoon baking powder

3 tablespoons chilled
   butter
6 to 8 tablespoons skim
   milk, divided

Preheat oven to 425°F. Spray a baking sheet with vegetable spray.

In a medium-size bowl, whisk together whole wheat pastry flour, unbleached white flour, and baking powder. Cut in butter with a pastry blender until mixture is crumbly.

With a wooden spoon, stir in ¼ cup of the skim milk. Add more milk, 1 tablespoon at a time, until dough clings together. Divide dough into 6 pieces and drop onto prepared baking sheet. Bake on middle shelf of oven for 10 minutes.

Remove to wire racks to cool.

Makes 6 servings
(132 calories per serving)

Vanilla Ice Milk

⅓ cup honey
1 vanilla bean
1 tablespoon vanilla extract
1 quart low-fat milk, divided

In a medium-size saucepan, mix together honey, vanilla bean, vanilla extract, and 1 cup of the low-fat milk. Add remaining low-fat milk and heat to scalding, stirring occasionally. Remove from heat and let stand 20 to 30 minutes. Remove vanilla bean.

Process mixture in an ice cream maker according to manufacturer's instructions, or turn mixture into a large pan and place in freezer until partially frozen. Remove from freezer, beat to break down ice crystals, and then return to freezer. Repeat this procedure twice, turning mixture into 2 1-quart containers the last time. Freeze until ready to serve.

Makes about 8 servings
(115 calories per serving)

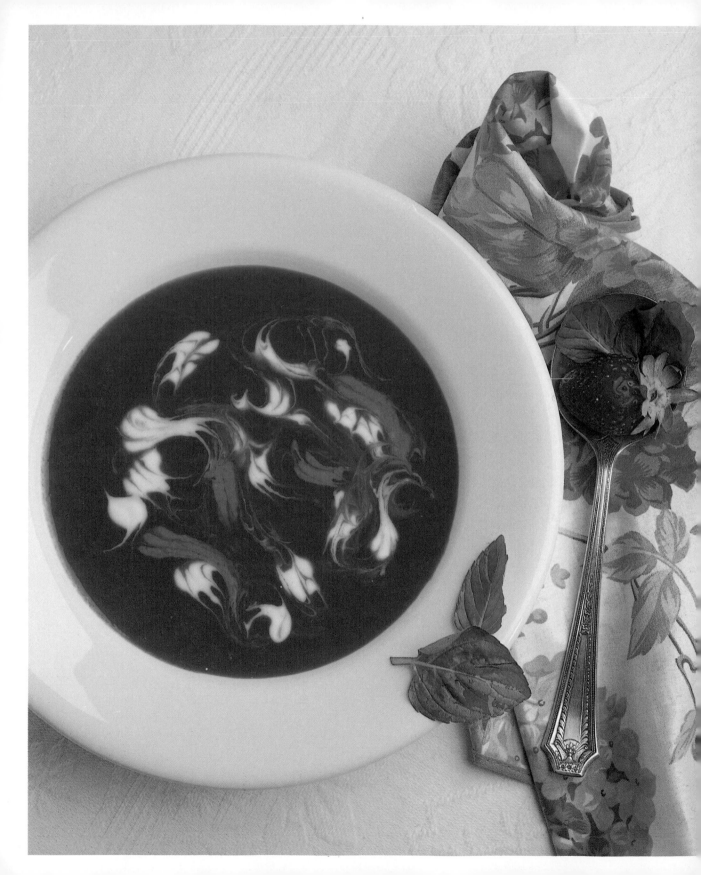

Good Old Strawberry Shortcake

3 cups fresh strawberries,
   quartered
2 tablespoons maple syrup
6 Skinny Shortcakes (page 79)
1 cup plain low-fat yogurt, divided

Combine strawberries with maple syrup in a large bowl and chill for 2 hours. Toss again after 1 hour to coat all berries.

Split shortcakes crosswise. Divide berries among shortcakes, piling them on bottom halves. Put tops of shortcakes over berries. Top each with 2 tablespoons of the yogurt. Serve immediately.

Makes 6 servings
(197 calories per serving)

Old-Fashioned Custard

4 eggs
3 tablespoons honey
2 cups skim milk
1½ teaspoons vanilla extract
   ground nutmeg for sprinkling

Preheat oven to 325°F. Spray 6 custard cups or a 6-cup glass casserole with vegetable spray.

In a large bowl, beat together eggs and honey until light colored. Beat in remaining ingredients. Divide among prepared custard cups, or pour into casserole. Put into a shallow pan on middle shelf of oven. Pour hot water into pan until it almost reaches the tops of the custard cups or casserole. Bake until a knife inserted into centers of custards comes out almost clean, 45 to 60 minutes.

Sprinkle with nutmeg and serve warm or chilled.

Makes 6 servings
(116 calories per serving)

Cool Strawberry Soup (page 77)

Carob Confections

⅓ cup butter
¼ cup carob chips
2 eggs
¼ cup honey
1 teaspoon vanilla extract
¼ cup whole wheat pastry flour
¼ cup unbleached white flour
½ cup Easy Vanilla Frosting
    (page 12)
2 tablespoons unsweetened flaked
    coconut

Preheat oven to 350°F.

In the top of a double boiler set over boiling water, melt together butter and carob chips. Set aside to cool.

In a medium-size bowl, beat together eggs, honey, and vanilla. Stir in carob mixture. In a small bowl, mix whole wheat pastry flour and unbleached white flour together with a whisk and then stir into carob mixture with a spoon until well blended. Turn into an 8 × 8-inch pan with a nonstick surface and bake on middle shelf of oven for 20 to 25 minutes, or until batter pulls away from sides of pan. If bubbles form in the middle, push them down with the back of a spatula.

When cool, spread frosting on top and sprinkle with coconut. Cut into 32 pieces.

Makes 16 servings
(100 calories per serving)

Peanut Butter Drop Cookies

⅔ cup whole wheat pastry flour
⅓ cup unbleached white flour
1 teaspoon baking powder
3 tablespoons butter, softened
¼ cup Reduced Calorie Peanut
    Butter (page 59)
2 tablespoons maple syrup
2 tablespoons honey
1 teaspoon vanilla extract
1 egg

Preheat oven to 350°F.

In a medium-size bowl, sift together whole wheat pastry flour, unbleached white flour, and baking powder. Whisk to blend well.

In a large bowl, beat together butter and peanut butter until fluffy. Beat in maple syrup, honey, vanilla, and egg. Mix dry ingredients into peanut butter mixture, blending well. Drop by tablespoonfuls onto 2 nonstick baking sheets and bake each batch on middle shelf of oven for 8 minutes.

Makes 3 dozen cookies
(36 calories per cookie)

Apricot Brandy Ice

There's something really refreshing about a fruit ice on a hot day.

> 2 **cups water**
> 3 **cups peeled, pitted fresh apricots**
> ½ **cup honey**
> 1½ **teaspoons brandy extract**

In a large saucepan, bring water to a boil. Add apricots, reduce heat, and poach until soft, about 10 minutes. Drain well, reserving juice, and set aside to cool.

In a food processor, puree apricots. Add 2 cups of the reserved apricot juice and remaining ingredients and process until blended.

Process mixture in an ice cream maker according to manufacturer's instructions, or put mixture into a large, shallow pan and place in freezer until thickened but not solid. Remove from freezer, beat to break down ice crystals, and then return to freezer. Repeat this procedure twice, spooning mixture into a container the last time. Freeze until ready to serve.

Makes 8 servings
(94 calories per serving)

Happy Easter Baskets

Both children and adults love these festive dessert baskets.

> 2 **recipes for Meringue Shells (page 84)**
> 2 **cups Raspberry Rum Sherbet (page 165)**
> 2 **cups French Carob Ice Milk (page 198) or Vanilla Ice Milk (page 79)**
> 1½ **cups Slim Pastry Cream (page 270), divided**
> ½ **cup unsweetened flaked coconut, divided**

Bake Meringue Shells according to directions.

Line a baking sheet with waxed paper. With the large end of a melon baller, scoop out balls of Raspberry Rum Sherbet and put them on prepared baking sheet. Do the same with French Carob Ice Milk or Vanilla Ice Milk. Place in freezer until serving time.

Put 2 tablespoons of the pastry cream into each meringue shell. Top with 2 of each kind of frozen balls. Sprinkle each with 1½ teaspoons of the coconut and serve immediately.

Makes 12 servings
(129 calories per serving)

Meringue Shells

*These shells make a wonderful base for many desserts,
and they always add a note of elegance.*

4 egg whites
¼ teaspoon cream of tartar

2 teaspoons maple syrup
1 teaspoon vanilla extract

Preheat oven to 250°F. Butter and lightly flour a large baking sheet.

In a large bowl, beat egg whites until foamy. Add cream of tartar and continue beating, drizzling in maple syrup and vanilla, until stiff peaks form.

Divide beaten egg whites into 6 mounds, evenly spacing them on prepared baking sheet. With the back of a spoon, flatten mounds slightly and make large indentations in centers. Bake on middle shelf of oven until golden, 40 to 50 minutes.

Carefully remove from baking sheet with a spatula and cool on wire racks.

Makes 6 servings
(15 calories per serving)

Very Vanilla Pudding

2 cups skim milk, divided
3 tablespoons cornstarch
2 tablespoons honey
1 teaspoon butter
1 egg, beaten
1 tablespoon vanilla extract

In the top of a double boiler set over boiling water, heat 1½ cups of the skim milk.

Shake remaining skim milk and cornstarch together in a jar with a tight-fitting lid. Add gradually to milk, mixing well. Stir in honey and continue to cook, stirring constantly, until mixture thickens. Stir in butter until melted. Mix a small amount of hot mixture into egg. Pour back into hot mixture and continue cooking, stirring constantly, for another 2 minutes. Remove from heat and stir in vanilla.

Makes 4 servings
(127 calories per serving)

Applesauce Fluff

2 cups unsweetened Applesauce
    (page 90), divided
2 egg whites
⅛ teaspoon cream of tartar
1 tablespoon honey
½ teaspoon ground cinnamon

Preheat oven to 425°F.
Put ½ cup of the applesauce in each of 4 custard cups.

In a medium-size bowl, beat egg whites until foamy. Add cream of tartar, honey, and cinnamon. Beat until stiff peaks form.

Divide among custard cups, spreading to cover Applesauce. Bake on middle shelf of oven until meringue is golden brown, about 5 minutes.

Makes 4 servings
(75 calories per serving)

Peach Soufflé

2 envelopes unflavored gelatin
½ cup cold water
1 20-ounce package unsweetened
    frozen peaches, thawed
¼ cup maple syrup
2 tablespoons honey
2 teaspoons vanilla extract

3 egg whites
¼ teaspoon cream of tartar
1 cup evaporated skim milk,
    chilled
2 tablespoons currant jelly

Fit a 2-quart soufflé dish with a soufflé collar.*

In a small saucepan, sprinkle gelatin over cold water. Set aside for 5 minutes to soften. Heat over medium heat, stirring constantly, until gelatin dissolves. Remove from heat.

In a food processor, puree peaches with maple syrup, honey, vanilla, and gelatin. Chill until thickened but not set. Whisk until smooth.

In a medium-size bowl, beat egg whites until foamy. Add cream of tartar and continue beating until stiff. Fold in peach mixture.

In a large bowl, beat evaporated skim milk to the consistency of whipped cream. Fold into peach mixture. Turn peach mixture into soufflé dish and chill until firm.

In a small saucepan, melt jelly. Drizzle over soufflé and return to refrigerator. Remove collar before serving.

Makes 12 servings
(94 calories per serving)

*To make a soufflé collar, cut a piece of foil 10 inches wide and long enough to encircle the soufflé dish plus 2 inches. Fold lengthwise. Tie collar around dish with string, allowing the foil to extend 3 inches above the rim. Tape the seam together. Butter or oil inside of collar.

Carob Crumb Apples

I like this dessert. It's an unlikely delightful blending of flavors.

    4 apples, peeled, cored, and
          chopped
    2 teaspoons freshly squeezed
          lemon juice
    ¼ cup honey
    ⅓ cup plus 3 tablespoons whole
          wheat pastry flour, divided
    1 teaspoon ground cinnamon
    ½ cup carob chips
    2 tablespoons butter
    ⅓ cup unbleached white flour

Preheat oven to 350°F. Spray a 9-inch pie plate with vegetable spray.

In a large bowl, toss apples with lemon juice, honey, 3 tablespoons of the whole wheat pastry flour, and cinnamon. Turn into prepared pie plate and bake on middle shelf of oven for 25 minutes.

In the top of a double boiler set over hot water, melt together carob chips and butter. Remove from heat.

In a small bowl, whisk remaining whole wheat pastry flour and unbleached white flour to blend. Stir into carob mixture. The mixture will separate into crumbs. Distribute crumbs evenly over top of apple mixture and return to oven for 25 minutes. Serve warm.

Makes 10 servings
(159 calories per serving)

Strawberry Grape Pie

    3 cups fresh strawberries, quartered
    2 cups seedless white grapes,
          halved
    ¼ cup cornstarch
    1 teaspoon vanilla extract
    ½ teaspoon brandy extract,
          optional
    2 tablespoons honey
    1 recipe for Skinny Piecrust
          (page 6)

Preheat oven to 400°F. Spray a 9-inch pie plate with vegetable spray.

In a large bowl, toss together strawberries, grapes, cornstarch, vanilla, and brandy extract, if desired. Add honey and toss to coat. Turn into prepared pie plate.

Roll out piecrust into a 10 × 6-inch piece. Cut into 4 1½-inch strips and make a spoke pattern on top of filling. Bake on middle shelf of oven until pastry is browned and filling bubbly, about 30 minutes.

Allow to cool before serving.

Makes 10 servings
(105 calories per serving)

Fluffy Almond Tapioca (page 89)

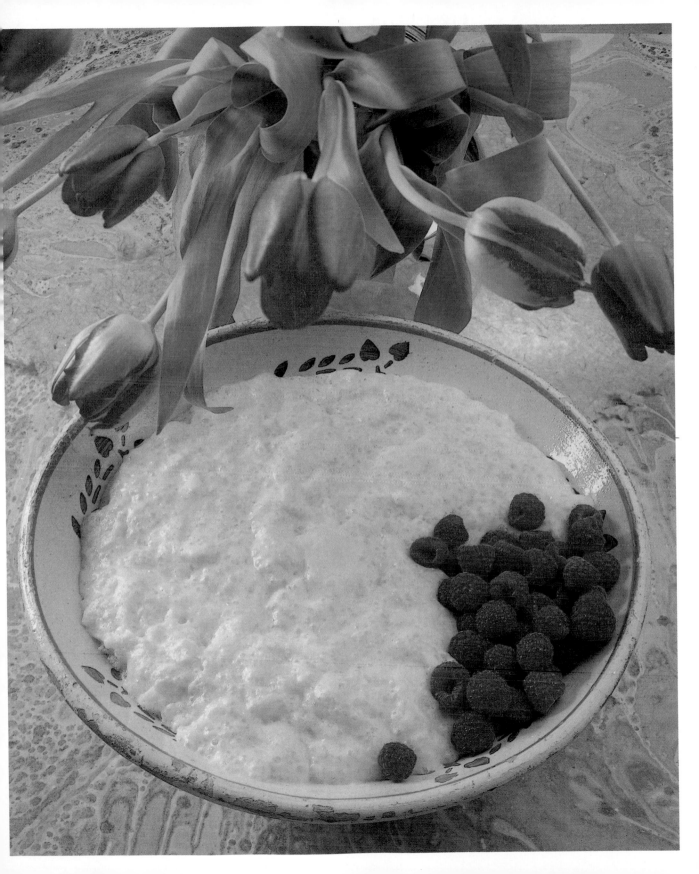

Piña Colada Pie

1 tablespoon cornstarch
2 cups skim milk, divided
2 envelopes unflavored gelatin,
   divided
2 tablespoons honey, divided
½ teaspoon vanilla extract
1 teaspoon rum extract, divided
½ cup unsweetened flaked coconut
1 20-ounce can unsweetened
   crushed pineapple

Spray a 9-inch pie plate with vegetable spray.

In a medium-size saucepan, dissolve cornstarch in 1 cup of the skim milk. Sprinkle 1 envelope of the gelatin over milk and set aside for 5 minutes to soften. Add 1 tablespoon of the honey and heat over medium heat, stirring constantly, until mixture thickens and gelatin dissolves. Stir in vanilla, ½ teaspoon of the rum extract, remaining skim milk, and coconut. Pour into prepared pie plate and chill until set, about 2 hours.

Drain pineapple, collecting juice in a small saucepan. Sprinkle remaining gelatin over juice and set aside for 5 minutes to soften. Heat over medium heat, stirring constantly, until gelatin dissolves. Remove from heat and stir in remaining honey and remaining rum extract. Mix into pineapple and let cool slightly. Spread over coconut mixture and chill until set.

Makes 8 servings
(144 calories per serving)

Almond Yogurt

1 envelope unflavored gelatin
½ cup water
1 cup plain low-fat yogurt
¼ cup honey
2 teaspoons vanilla extract
1 teaspoon almond extract
¾ cup evaporated skim milk,
   chilled
1 kiwi fruit, sliced

In a small saucepan, sprinkle gelatin over water and set aside for 5 minutes to soften. Heat over medium heat, stirring constantly, until gelatin dissolves.

In a medium-size bowl, combine yogurt, honey, and extracts. Fold in gelatin and refrigerate until thickened but not set, about 30 minutes.

In a large bowl, beat evaporated skim milk to the consistency of whipped cream. Fold in yogurt mixture and divide among 8 dessert glasses. Chill until set.

Decorate with kiwi slices and serve.

Makes 8 servings
(84 calories per serving)

Strawberry Bread Pudding

Fresh strawberries produce a firmer, more satisfactory dessert, but the recipe will work with frozen berries if they're drained well.

2 cups skim milk
⅓ cup honey
1 teaspoon butter
2 eggs
1 teaspoon vanilla extract
1 teaspoon brandy extract
2 cups cubed fresh whole grain bread (4 or 5 slices)
1 cup coarsely chopped fresh strawberries
2 egg whites
⅛ teaspoon cream of tartar

Preheat oven to 350°F. Spray a 1½-quart casserole with vegetable spray.

In a large saucepan, heat skim milk and honey together to scalding. Remove from heat, mix in butter, and set aside to cool slightly.

In a small bowl, beat eggs. Whisk into cooled milk along with extracts. Stir in bread and strawberries.

In a medium-size bowl, beat egg whites until foamy. Add cream of tartar and continue beating until stiff but not dry. Fold into other ingredients.

Turn into prepared casserole and place in a pan of hot water on middle shelf of oven. Bake until a knife inserted about 1 inch from center comes out clean, 50 to 60 minutes. Center will cook after pudding has been removed from oven. Serve warm or cold.

Makes 8 servings
(141 calories per serving)

Fluffy Almond Tapioca

3 tablespoons quick-cooking tapioca
3 tablespoons honey, divided
2 cups skim milk
1 egg, separated
½ teaspoon vanilla extract
½ teaspoon almond extract

In a medium-size saucepan, combine tapioca, 2 tablespoons of the honey, and skim milk. Beat egg yolk, add to mixture, and set aside for 5 minutes to soften tapioca.

In a small bowl, beat egg white until stiff peaks form, drizzling in the remaining honey and extracts.

Bring softened tapioca mixture to a boil, stirring constantly. Reduce heat and continue cooking, stirring constantly, for 6 minutes. Set aside to cool for about 10 minutes and then fold in beaten egg white. Serve warm or cold.

Makes 5 servings
(121 calories per serving)

Cottage Cheese Pie

½ tablespoon butter or margarine
3 tablespoons graham cracker
   crumbs
¼ teaspoon ground cinnamon
16 ounces low-fat, cream-style
   cottage cheese
4 teaspoons cornstarch
¼ cup honey
1½ teaspoons vanilla extract
1 teaspoon freshly squeezed
   lemon juice
2 eggs
10 fresh strawberries, halved

Preheat oven to 350°F.
Rinse an 8½-inch glass pie plate in hot water. Dry well and rub butter on bottom of pie plate until all the butter is used. Sprinkle with graham cracker crumbs and press lightly to make crust.

Put remaining ingredients, except strawberries, into a food processor or blender and blend until smooth. Pour over crust and bake on middle shelf of oven until set, about 30 minutes.

Cool well, then decorate with strawberry halves.

Makes 10 servings
(102 calories per serving)

Strawberry Fizz

1 cup fresh or unsweetened frozen
   strawberries, thawed
2 teaspoons honey
1 teaspoon vanilla extract
½ cup club soda

In a blender, puree strawberries with honey and vanilla. Stir in club soda. Pour over ice in individual glasses and serve immediately.

Makes 2 servings
(48 calories per serving)

Mango Strawberry Crepe Stacks

1 cup evaporated skim milk,
   chilled
1 tablespoon honey
½ teaspoon vanilla extract
½ cup Slim Pastry Cream (page 270)
2 cups diced mangoes
2 cups quartered fresh
   strawberries
8 Delicious Diet Crepes (page 33)

In a large bowl, beat evaporated skim milk until foamy. Drizzle in honey and vanilla and continue beating just until soft peaks form. Fold in pastry cream and fruit.

Place 1 crepe on a large plate. Spread about ⅐th of the fruit mixture on it. Put another crepe on top. Continue making layers, ending with a crepe. Slice, like a cake, with a serrated knife and serve immediately, or whipped milk will lose its volume.

Makes 8 servings
(155 calories per serving)

Frozen Bananas

2 large, firm bananas
1 tablespoon freshly squeezed
   lemon juice
2 tablespoons honey, warmed
2 tablespoons Coconut Sugar
   (page 66)

Line a baking sheet with waxed paper.

Cut bananas into halves, crosswise, and brush lightly with lemon juice to prevent darkening. Insert popsicle sticks into cut ends of banana halves. Brush honey on all surfaces of bananas. Roll in Coconut Sugar, place on prepared baking sheet, and freeze until firm. Wrap individually and return to freezer.

Makes 4 servings
(72 calories per serving)

MAY

Selecting Fresh Fruit, the Dieter's Ally

				1	2	3
FRUIT OF THE MONTH: **BLUEBERRIES** *DESSERT OF THE MONTH:* **BLUEBERRY ICE MILK** *DRINK OF THE MONTH:* **COMPANY PUNCH**				BLUEBERRIES WITH MAPLE YOGURT	LIGHT COFFEE SOUFFLÉ	PINEAPPLE SNOW
4 SKINNY PEACH PUDDING	5 STRAWBERRY BLISS	6 BLUEBERRY ICE MILK ★	7 PRUNE CUPCAKES	*Mother's Day* 8 CARNATION CASSATA	9 SPRING DOVE	10 RUBY RED GRANITA
11 LOVELY LEMON SQUARES	12 BLUEBERRY TANGERINE PIE	13 PAPAYA FLUFF	14 TAPIOCA PARFAITS	15 ORANGE PUDDING	16 PURPLE POPS	17 PEACHY RASPBERRY TORTE
18 LIME CHIFFON PIE	19 ½ CUP FRESH BLUEBERRIES WITH ¼ CUP SKIM MILK	20 STRAWBERRY PECAN CREPE ROLLS	21 MANGO YOGURT PUDDING	22 BANANA SMOOTHIES	23 LITE MERINGUE KISSES	24 PRUNE CONFECTIONS
25 BANANA STRAWBERRY FREEZE	26 PAPAYA LAYER CAKE	27 APPLESAUCE MERINGUE	28 STRAWBERRY PEACH PIE	29 PAPAYA BASKETS	*Memorial Day* 30 CRUSTLESS BLUEBERRY CHEESECAKE	31 STRAWBERRY RHUBARB PIE WITH MERINGUE CRUST

Papaya Fluff (page 120)

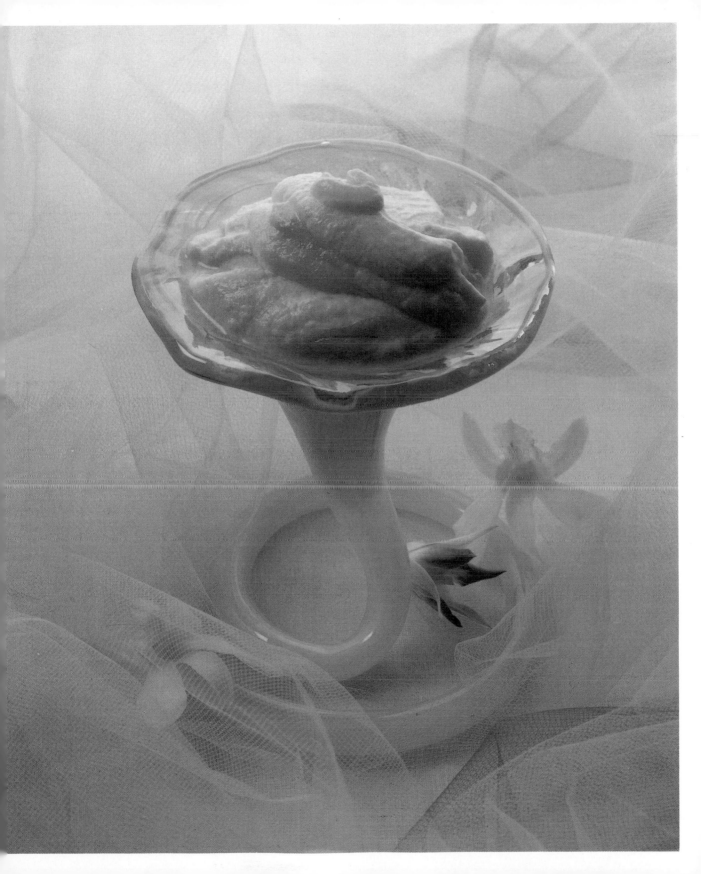

$\mathcal{T}$he beauty of fruit for the dieter is that it's nutritious and mostly low calorie, it makes you feel full due to its high fiber content, and some kinds are available in the markets during every month of the year. Add to all that the natural sweetness it imparts to desserts and you have a near-perfect diet food.

Selecting fruits at their succulent best can mean the difference between creating a superior dessert and one that's just so-so. While some fruits are always abundant, each fruit has a special season, and that's when its quality excels. Happily, when a fruit is truly in season, it is also least expensive.

Choosing fruit is an art you can learn. Your eyes, nose, and fingers are all good indicators of the quality of a piece of fruit—don't be afraid to use them. A superior specimen adds so much to the finished dish, especially when fruit is used raw.

Purchase ripe fruit close to the time you're planning to use it. With few exceptions, such as citrus fruits and apples, fruit is delicate and wilts quickly. If you're buying unripe fruit, you need to know how long it will take to ripen so you can plan its use. Don't be tempted by sale fruit that's past its prime unless you're planning to make jam or preserves. Even then, by the time you've cut out all the bruised and spoiled spots, you may find you've actually paid more per pound than you would have for top quality.

Individual Fruits and What You Should Know about Them

Here are some fruits I use often in making desserts with tips on how to select, ripen, and store them so they can be enjoyed at top quality.

Apples: One of America's favorite fruits, apples are available year round.

They range from fiery red to the palest of yellows—from sugary sweet to lemony sour. The type of apple you select depends entirely on how you intend to use it. For instance, those wonderfully sweet, Red Delicious apples are a delight to sink your teeth into, living up to their name, but they're not good for cooking.

Look for apples that have good color for their variety and unbroken, unbruised skins. Bruises indicate that the fruit has been subjected to freezing temperatures, which apples can't withstand. Scald (tan or brown spots so common on apples) affects only the portion of apple where it occurs; just cut out and discard the affected part.

Handle each apple before you buy, if possible. It should feel uniformly firm, not mushy or soft in spots. Soft apples have a mealy texture; you want crispness.

Although there are many wonderful varieties of tart apples for cooking, I usually opt for a sweet apple in cooking desserts. This cuts down on the sweetener necessary to produce a delectable dessert. The bright red Cortland is one of my favorites for pies. The York apple with its light red background speckled with russet is a marvelous all-around cooking apple that, because of its firmness, retains its shape—not disintegrating as some juicier apples do during cooking. The Winesap, while slightly less sweet than the other two, is an excellent pie apple. But use a trifle more thickener than you do with Yorks since Winesaps are very juicy apples. Golden Delicious are also firm, and I favor them for cooking.

Apples that aren't fully mature before picking lack both flavor and color. Don't rely on time to ripen them. It won't happen.

If you're buying apples in the net bags in which they're so frequently sold, avoid any labeled U.S. No. 2—they're a low grade. Instead look for U.S. Extra Fancy, U.S. Fancy, or U.S. No. 1.

Apples will keep in a cool place or in the refrigerator during hot weather. Heat wilts them prematurely. But in the right environment, apples stay useable for several weeks, although they may become rather lackluster after a week or two. Don't store them near vegetables; apples give off ethylene gas which causes many vegetables to spoil.

Apricots: This ancient fruit with a distinctive flavor has been grown in California since 1792 and dates back to before the birth of Christ.

If you've ever bitten into an apricot and found it startlingly sour, you've eaten one that was picked before it had a chance to mature. Immature apricots have a greenish tinge. Avoid them; they'll never be good eating! Plump flesh of golden-orange fruit, yielding to slight pressure without feeling mushy, is the hallmark of an apricot at its best. A yellow rather than golden hue signals an over-mature specimen.

Utah and Washington State now vie with California for the apricot trade. And among them they keep the markets of our country supplied with apricots during June and July. If selected at its peak, this lovely fruit will keep for a couple of days wrapped tightly in plastic and refrigerated.

Avocados: Yes, avocados are high in calories, but they're also delicious and, unlike other fruits, contain iron and protein. So I occasionally use avocado with a mixture of caution and other lower-calorie ingredients — quite sparingly.

There's no readily discernible difference between the flavor of the Fuerte (winter avocado) and the Haas (summer avocado). Black or purple spots are a sign of decay on either variety as are cracked or broken skins. Avocados must be fully ripe before they're used. A ripe avocado is almost squishy soft. Allow firm fruit to ripen for three to five days at room temperature. If you purchase a fully ripe avocado and don't wish to use it immediately, store it, unwrapped, in the refrigerator.

Bananas: There's a lot to be said for bananas: most people like them, they know no season, and they're good diet fare.

While most fruit should be harvested when fully ripe, bananas are always picked green. They do much of their ripening in transit to our markets. As they ripen, bananas turn from green to yellow. When the fruit becomes flecked with brown and softens to the touch, it's perfect for use. Dark brown patches indicate overripe bananas — undesirable for either eating or cooking as the flesh is usually dark brown, too.

Chiquita Banana notwithstanding, to keep a ripe banana from going bad, store it in the refrigerator for a day or so. This may cause the skin to darken, but it will preserve the flesh of the fruit. But an unripe banana must be stored at room temperature — the chill of the refrigerator will halt its ripening process permanently.

Blueberries: May through September is blueberry season. And if you're lucky enough to live in an area where you can go blueberry picking, you know the glorious flavor of freshly picked berries, eaten plain or with a bit of milk or cream. But the rest of us, who rely on the local market or farmstand, must select berries cautiously.

Fresh blueberries picked at their prime, have a dark blue color touched with a silverish coating. The bloom, as this coating is called, isn't a spray, but a natural phenomenon protecting the freshness of the berries. Blueberries should be plump with dry skins, free of slime. No stems or leaves should be in the basket you select. Keep blueberries in the refrigerator for no more than three days lightly covered, so they can breathe.

Cantaloupes (Muskmelons): This familiar low-calorie melon has a strong flavor. Cantaloupes should ripen on the vine; they separate from their stems when fully ripe. Unfortunately, they're often picked prematurely. Look for a small indentation at the stem end that's well-formed and smooth. If a melon is picked too early, the indentation has a ragged appearance, indicating the fruit was ripped from the stem.

The netting on a cantaloupe should stand out from the rest of the surface and be coarse and well defined. The color underneath the netting shouldn't be green, but rather light yellowish, gray, or tan. A green melon won't ripen, but it will rot. If the color under the netting is a bright yellow, the melon is overripe.

Your nose is an invaluable resource in selecting melons. When a cantaloupe reaches its peak of ripeness, it has a strong but pleasant melonlike aroma. Then it's best for eating. A day later it will be overripe. The blossom end of a ripe cantaloupe yields to slight pressure.

Cantaloupes flood the markets from May through September. A ripe one can be kept, tightly wrapped, in the refrigerator for a couple of days, but the aroma is so strong it may taint some of your other foods, so keep it away from butter and like items. Hold unripe cantaloupe at room temperature until the blossom end is soft.

Cherries: Can you bake a cherry pie and stay on a diet? The answer is a definite yes! But while cherry pies are traditionally made with sour cherries, I use the sweeter varieties to avoid having to load the pies with sweeteners.

When you're shopping for cherries keep in mind that the darker fruit is sweeter. Bing, Black Tartarian, Chapman, Lambert, and Schmidt are all acceptable varieties. Cherries should have their stems intact (they help keep the fruit fresh), and the stems should look bright and alive rather than dried out. A healthy cherry is fat and glossy with no signs of brown spots or leaking skin.

In most places you'll find cherries on the market from May through August, but they're best and most plentiful in June and July.

Cherries are highly perishable. They should be stored in a basket or other airy container, uncovered, with stems still on and used as soon as possible—ideally the day of purchase, but certainly within two days.

Cranberries: The little red berry that conjures up visions of Pilgrims, Thanksgiving, and turkey is also a tasty ingredient for desserts. Unfortunately, cranberries are usually sold in sealed plastic bags bearing printed information, which makes it almost impossible to tell what the berries look like. But if you're lucky enough to find berries that aren't packaged this way, look for firm, plump berries with shiny skins. Most varieties are dark red when ripe, but there are some that have a bright red skin. Shun any soft berries. They'll be sour and give your recipe an "off" taste.

Cranberries are plentiful from September through January, although you'll find the supply at its peak during November and December.

Lightly covered and refrigerated, they'll keep for several weeks.

Grapefruits: What experienced dieter isn't familiar with this citrus fruit? It's as much a staple of dieting as cottage cheese.

The pink varieties are sweeter than the more traditional yellow. Whichever color you prefer, look for fruit that feels firm and heavy for its size. Although the fruit should be uniformly firm, it also should have a slightly spongy feeling when pressed. This sponginess indicates a thin skin and a juicy flesh. If the stem end of the grapefruit is pointed, the skin is thick and the fruit won't be as juicy. A mottled skin with uneven color has no bearing on the quality of the fruit inside.

This good source of vitamins A and C is available year round but is in greatest abundance January through May.

Grapefruits keep nicely in the refrigerator for several weeks.

Grapes: Seedless Thompson grapes are the most popular and the ones you'll find in greatest abundance in the markets. They're sweeter and a bit higher in calories than other grape varieties, such as the Concord, so you may wonder why I use them so often in my diet recipes. The answer is simple—they don't need added sweetener as do some other types of grapes.

When selecting grapes, look for healthy-appearing, greenish stems, bearing firm-fleshed fruit. Green grapes should be yellow tinged, while darker varieties should have an even color. Leaking or wrinkled grapes are past their prime so pass them by.

These little gems are available all year. They're quite perishable but will keep, uncovered, in the refrigerator for about three days.

Honeydew Melons: Slightly higher in calories than the cantaloupe, the milder tasting honeydew is nonetheless worthy of a place in the menu of a dieter. The season for honeydews goes from June through October. Although a few can be found in the other months, they'll be of poor quality.

Look for honeydew with smooth, white to yellow skins—never greenish—with only slight netting. Store them as you would cantaloupes (page 99).

Kiwi Fruits (Chinese Gooseberries): This Johnny-come-lately to the American marketplace has become a favorite in fruit salads and as a garnish, but it's a useful addition to desserts as well. I've seen kiwis in the local markets all year, but I find the summer fruit far more desirable.

The kiwi's brown, fuzzy surface yields to slight pressure when the fruit is ripe. The bright green flesh, flecked with tiny, black, edible seeds, has a flavor that suggests a mixture of strawberry, pineapple, and papaya. A ripe kiwi will keep in the refrigerator, uncovered, for about three days.

Lemons: From California and Arizona come enough lemons to keep the country supplied year round with this tart, useful fruit. When lemons are their fresh best, they sport smooth, blemish-free, bright yellow skins. A pale yellow or greenish skin holds an acceptable, although slightly inferior, lemon. But dark yellow or hard skins are certain indications the fruit is dried out and tasteless.

Since lemons are so plentiful, there's no reason to settle for inferior fruit, ever.

Lemons keep well for about two weeks when stored in a refrigerator. I always use freshly squeezed lemon juice in my recipes. Even if it's only a tablespoon or two, the difference between fresh and bottled is monumental.

Limes: Used almost interchangeably with lemons by many cooks, the lime is deserving of a place of its own in the culinary world.

Most of the limes commonly found in our markets are Persian or Tahitian limes. At its best this fruit is bright green and glossy. A purplish-brown spot on the skin, scald, is undesirable only in an advanced stage.

Key limes, which are far more difficult to come by in most parts of the country, are greenish yellow and, of course, are the main ingredients of the famous key lime pie. Although you'll find limes year round, during the winter months you may have to search to find respectable ones. They'll keep for about two weeks stored, uncovered, in the refrigerator or in a cool room.

Mangoes: A fairly recent gift to us from the tropics, mangoes are ready for use when their skins are green with yellow or red areas. They will yield to slight pressure. You'll find mangoes in plenty from May through August. You can keep them in the refrigerator for a maximum of three days.

Nectarines: Don't buy nectarines that are shriveled or have cracked skin. The fully ripe, ideal nectarine yields to pressure along the indentation but the skin stays intact. If it's past its prime, you'll find the fruit leaky when pressed.

If you don't intend to use nectarines for a few days, purchase hard ones and allow them to ripen at room temperature. Ripe nectarines will hold their quality for a day or so in the refrigerator.

Although June and July are the best months for nectarines, you'll find them in the markets in August and September as well.

Oranges: What would we do without the sunshine fruit? It adds flavor to pies, cakes, puddings, and the juice is a healthy thirst quencher and useful ingredient in so many desserts. To top it off, the orange is available year round.

Oranges should feel heavy for their size and be firm to the touch. Pineapple and Navel oranges are good eating, while Parson Browns and Hamlins are better juicers.

The skin color of oranges covers the spectrum from greenish orange to a mottled orange with white or golden spots. Russeting, those tan to black spots you see on Florida or Texas oranges, is a sign of thin skin and good quality. Many oranges are dyed an even orange color and should be so labeled.

I never buy oranges in bags, preferring to select each fruit individually, handling it and making sure I have the best there is to offer. Bags are admittedly cheaper, but the few times I've succumbed to the lure of a good buy, I've found at least one rotten orange in the bag.

Oranges keep well for several weeks in the refrigerator.

Papayas: I just love this fruit with its naturally sweet, juicy goodness and flavor that's a cross between a cantaloupe and a peach. But I limit my use of them to May and June when they're most abundant and least expensive. However, if you wish to eat papayas in January, you'll probably find them in your local market.

Whatever season you buy them, look for yellow, greenish yellow, or green and yellow fruit that yields to gentle pressure. Ripe papayas keep for up to two days in the refrigerator.

Peaches: Of the two varieties of peaches, Freestone is what you're more apt to find in the market. Clingstone, the other type, has stones that cling stubbornly to the flesh and is used mostly for canning. The skin of a peach, may be either fuzzy or smooth, although the smooth variety has gained in popularity. A healthy ripe fruit is yellow or cream-colored with red areas. If a peach is green, don't buy it. It was picked before maturity and will never ripen. Bruised peaches are a poor choice no matter how much of a bargain they seem. They spoil very quickly.

July and August are the prime "peachy" months, but this fruit is available May through September.

Keep ripe peaches in the refrigerator and use them within a day or two. Leave unripened peaches at room temperature for a day or two and they'll ripen nicely.

Pears: Among the many varieties of this fruit, Bartletts are the most common. Pears are stubborn about ripening and purchasing them with this expectation is usually doomed to failure. You'll most often end up with rotten rather than ripe fruit. Instead, choose ripe pears that yield to soft pressure and have unblemished skins. They'll keep in your refrigerator for up to three days. Pears are available year round.

Persimmons: The plump persimmon is deep red with black flecks when ripe, but it can be purchased when it's yellowish orange and ripened at home. A ripe persimmon yields to pressure. Once ripe, the persimmon keeps well, uncovered, in the refrigerator for up to four days. This fruit will add to your dessert pleasure from October through November.

Pineapples: A pleasing aroma indicates a good ripe pineapple. If the odor is the least bit off, the pineapple has started to decay. Look for plump heavy fruit. Red Spanish and Smooth Cayeen are the two varieties in most American markets. When unripe they're green. A gorgeous orangy-yellow color emerges as the fruit ripens. A healthy pineapple has slightly separated eyes. Sunken eyes or bruises are signs of inferior fruit. Thanks to good transportation and improved storage, we can now enjoy pineapple year round.

Contrary to common opinion, pineapples should never be stored at room temperature. The Pineapple Growers' Association of Hawaii claims pineapple must be picked when ripe and will quickly ferment at room temperature. It will, however, keep for a week in the refrigerator. I believe they know what they're talking about, so I always keep fresh pineapple refrigerated, and with good success.

Plums: Did you ever bite into an unripe plum? They're so sour they make your lips pucker! Plums sweeten as they ripen, and no plum should be eaten before its time.

Though the color may range from red to purple, the skin should be even in color and unbroken. Leaky fruit is overripe fruit.

You'll find plums in abundance from June through September. What's offered during the winter months is, in my opinion, a poor excuse for the lush plum you'll get in season.

If plums aren't ripe when you buy them, a day or two at room temperature should do the trick. Then it's into the refrigerator, uncovered, where they'll stay fresh for another day or two.

Raspberries: One of the reasons I love summer is that it's raspberry season. From June through August, the luscious red berries are in great supply. But July is really raspberry month—the time when they're most abundant and the best eating.

Good red color and uniform size are indications of sweet eating berries. Although the small cells should look succulent, they shouldn't be leaking or mushy. These most marvelous of berries will keep in the refrigerator for a day or two (if you can resist them for that long).

Strawberries: I was delighted when I learned that strawberries would be available year round. Imagine fresh strawberry pie in January—what decadence! But I have found that the berries marketed in off months are over-large with a great deal of unappetizing white outside and very little juice or flavor inside. They're lifeless imitations of the real berries you'll find only from April to June.

Look for plump, red berries with bright green caps. If the caps are dried out, chances are the berries are too. Avoid leaking strawberries or those with mold. Examine the berries in the bottom of the basket as well.

Strawberries keep, lightly covered, in the refrigerator for up to three days.

Watermelons: I never buy a whole watermelon. It's virtually impossible to tell what secrets the green skin holds without cutting into it. I look for bright red, watery flesh with black or brown seeds and few, if any, white streaks. An immature melon has greenish seeds.

Watermelon, which is available May through September, will keep, covered, in the refrigerator for up to five days.

Unsweetened frozen fruit is a viable alternative when fresh fruit is out of season, and in many recipes the difference between frozen and fresh fruit is hardly discernible.

Most frozen fruit will keep for about ten months. To use it, thaw it in your refrigerator for eight to ten hours. Many people thaw frozen fruit at room temperature for about four hours. I'm not comfortable doing this and prefer the safer refrigerator method. And, of course, I never thaw anything under warm water! I do sometimes thaw fruit in my microwave, carefully following directions. And some recipes facilitate the use of frozen fruit without the bother of thawing it, particularly if the fruit is individually frozen, such as blueberries or strawberries, and can be removed from the package in separate pieces instead of in one large frozen mass.

Store all fresh fruit unwashed. Water hastens the decaying process. But do wash fruit well before using it.

Purple Pops

¾ cup milk
1 cup grape juice
¼ cup honey

Blend all ingredients in a blender. Divide among 8 2-ounce pop molds and freeze.

Makes 8 pops
(68 calories per pop)

Light Coffee Soufflé

This soufflé rises so high, it may push against the oven shelf above it. So I remove all shelves except the one on which the soufflé cooks.

2 tablespoons cornstarch
1½ teaspoons decaffeinated instant coffee
3 tablespoons honey
1 cup evaporated skim milk
2 teaspoons vanilla extract
½ teaspoon orange extract
6 egg whites
¼ teaspoon cream of tartar

Remove all but lower rack of oven. Preheat oven to 375°F. Fit a 2½-quart casserole or soufflé dish with a soufflé collar.*

In a large saucepan, blend together cornstarch and coffee. Mix in honey and skim milk, and cook over medium heat, stirring constantly, until mixture thickens. Remove from heat and stir in extracts.

In a large bowl, beat egg whites until foamy. Add cream of tartar and continue beating until stiff peaks form. Mix a small amount of beaten egg whites into coffee mixture to lighten. Fold in remaining whites and turn into prepared casserole or soufflé dish. (Or you may wish to use individual soufflé cups.) Bake for about 25 minutes (15 minutes for cups), or until soufflé has risen and is golden on top. Serve immediately.

Makes 8 servings
(69 calories per serving)

*To make a soufflé collar, cut a piece of foil 10 inches wide and long enough to encircle soufflé dish plus 2 inches. Fold lengthwise. Tie collar around dish with string, allowing foil to extend 3 inches above rim of dish. Tape seam together. Butter or oil inside of collar.

Skinny Peach Pudding

1½ envelopes unflavored gelatin
½ cup cold water
1 cup skim milk
3 tablespoons honey
4 cups ripe, peeled peaches
1 teaspoon almond extract

In a small saucepan, sprinkle gelatin over cold water and set aside to soften for 5 minutes. Add skim milk and honey and heat, stirring constantly, until milk is scalding.

In a food processor, puree peaches. Turn peach puree into a large bowl. Mix in milk mixture and almond extract. Divide among 8 dessert dishes and chill until set.

Makes 8 servings
(73 calories per serving)

Blueberries with Maple Yogurt

1 cup plain low-fat yogurt
3 tablespoons maple syrup
1 teaspoon vanilla extract
2 cups fresh blueberries

In a medium-size bowl, lightly mix together yogurt, maple syrup, and vanilla. Fold in blueberries and chill.

Makes 6 servings
(76 calories per serving)

Pineapple Snow

1 8-ounce can unsweetened
   crushed pineapple
2 teaspoons unflavored gelatin
1 tablespoon honey
½ teaspoon vanilla extract
1 egg white

Spray a 4-cup dessert mold with vegetable spray.

Drain pineapple, reserving juice. Add enough water to juice to make 1 cup.

In a medium-size saucepan, sprinkle gelatin over juice. Set aside for 5 minutes to soften. Mix in honey and heat, stirring, until gelatin is dissolved. Add vanilla and chill until thickened but not set, about 30 to 40 minutes.

In a medium-size bowl, beat egg white until stiff peaks form, then beat into thickened gelatin. Fold in pineapple and turn into mold.

Makes 4 servings
(83 calories per serving)

Prune Cupcakes

½ cup whole wheat pastry flour,
   divided
½ cup unbleached white flour
1 teaspoon baking powder
½ teaspoon ground cinnamon
¼ teaspoon ground nutmeg
¼ cup honey
½ cup prune juice
⅓ cup vegetable oil
1 egg
1 teaspoon vanilla extract
¼ cup prunes

Preheat oven to 350°F. Line 9 cups of a muffin tin with paper liners.

In a medium-size bowl, sift together all but 2 teaspoons of the whole wheat pastry flour, unbleached white flour, baking powder, cinnamon, and nutmeg. Whisk to blend. Mix in honey, prune juice, oil, egg, and vanilla. Beat for 3 minutes.

In a food processor, finely chop prunes with remaining whole wheat pastry flour. Fold into batter.

Divide among prepared muffin cups and bake on middle shelf of oven until a cake tester inserted into centers comes out clean, 20 to 25 minutes.

Remove from tin and cool on wire racks.

Makes 9 servings
(121 calories per serving)

Ladyfingers

This classic cake is an invaluable ingredient for many desserts.

3 eggs, separated
3 tablespoons honey
½ teaspoon vanilla extract
½ cup sifted whole wheat
   pastry flour

½ cup sifted unbleached
   white flour
1 tablespoon cornstarch
⅛ teaspoon cream of tartar

Preheat oven to 350°F. Line 2 baking sheets with parchment paper.

In a large bowl, beat egg yolks until golden. Add honey and beat for 10 minutes until ribbons form. Mix in vanilla.

Sift together whole wheat pastry flour, unbleached white flour, and cornstarch into a medium-size bowl. Whisk to blend. Fold flour mixture into egg mixture, a little at a time.

In a medium-size bowl, beat egg whites until foamy. Add cream of tartar and beat until stiff peaks form.

Fold beaten whites into batter. Put batter into pastry bag with ¾-inch opening. Squeeze 24 lengths of dough, about 3 inches long and about 1 inch apart, onto prepared baking sheets. Bake each batch on middle shelf of oven for 10 to 12 minutes, or until lightly browned.

Remove carefully with a spatula and cool on wire racks.

Makes 2 dozen fingers
(38 calories per finger)

Lite Meringue Kisses

Be sure to bake these meringues long enough for them to become dry. If they're underbaked they'll be sticky inside.

3 **egg whites**
⅛ **teaspoon cream of tartar**
¼ **cup maple syrup**
1 **teaspoon vanilla extract**

Preheat oven to 225°F. Line 2 baking sheets with parchment.

In a medium-size bowl, beat egg whites until foamy. Add cream of tartar and continue to beat, gradually adding maple syrup and vanilla, until whites are very stiff and dry.

Drop mixture by teaspoonfuls onto prepared baking sheets. Bake each batch on middle shelf of oven until lightly browned and dry, about 60 to 70 minutes.

Allow to cool before removing from baking sheet.

Makes 90 kisses
(3 calories per cookie)

Crustless Blueberry Cheesecake

2 **cups part-skim ricotta cheese**
3 **eggs**
2 **tablespoons cornstarch**
2 **tablespoons honey**
1 **teaspoon almond extract**
1 **teaspoon vanilla extract**
1½ **cups fresh blueberries**

Preheat oven to 325°F. Butter a 9-inch pie plate.

In a large bowl, beat ricotta and eggs together until smooth. Add cornstarch, honey, and extracts and beat just until blended. Turn into prepared pie plate and bake on middle shelf of oven for 1 hour.

Chill. Just before serving, top with blueberries.

Makes 8 servings
(160 calories per serving)

 ## Blueberry Ice Milk

3 **cups fresh blueberries**
⅓ **cup honey**
2 **cups skim milk**
1 **teaspoon vanilla extract**

In a medium-size saucepan, heat blueberries and honey to boiling, stirring constantly. Reduce heat and simmer for 10 minutes. Puree mixture in a blender. Strain pureed berries into a large bowl. Stir in skim milk and vanilla.

Process mixture in an ice cream maker according to manufacturer's instructions, or turn mixture into a pan, cover, and put in freezer until thickened but not frozen solid. Remove from freezer, beat to break down ice crystals, and then return to freezer. Repeat this procedure twice, putting ice milk into a covered container the last time before returning it to freezer. Freeze until ready to serve.

Makes 8 servings
(95 calories per serving)

Banana Smoothies

1 envelope unflavored gelatin
½ cup water
1⅓ cups cold water
⅔ cup nonfat dry milk
1 egg
2 tablespoons honey
2 teaspoons vanilla extract
2 bananas
    ground nutmeg for sprinkling,
        optional

In a small saucepan, sprinkle gelatin over water. Set aside for 5 minutes to soften. Heat over medium heat, stirring constantly, until gelatin dissolves.

Blend together cold water, nonfat dry milk, egg, honey, and vanilla in a blender. Add gelatin mixture and blend.

Cut bananas into small pieces, dividing them among 8 dessert dishes. Pour gelatin mixture on top and chill until set.

Sprinkle with nutmeg before serving, if desired.

Makes 8 servings
(90 calories per serving)

Lovely Lemon Squares

1 recipe for Skinny Piecrust
    (page 6)
2 eggs
⅓ cup honey
¼ cup whole wheat pastry flour
1 teaspoon baking powder
⅓ cup freshly squeezed lemon juice
½ teaspoon lemon extract

Preheat oven to 425°F. Spray an 8 × 8-inch pan with vegetable spray.

Roll piecrust into an 8-inch square. Place on bottom of prepared pan and bake blind on middle shelf of oven until lightly browned, about 10 minutes. Remove from oven and reduce heat to 350°F.

In a large bowl, slightly beat eggs and honey.

Sift together flour and baking powder into a small bowl. Whisk to blend. Beat into egg mixture. Beat in lemon juice and extract and pour over crust. Bake on middle shelf of oven for 20 minutes.

Cool in pan and cut into 9 squares.

Makes 9 servings
(135 calories per serving)

Blueberry Tangerine Pie

1 recipe for Mini Piecrust
    (page 113)
3 cups fresh or unsweetened
    frozen blueberries
2 tangerines, peeled and sectioned
3 tablespoons cornstarch
½ teaspoon ground cinnamon
½ cup honey

Preheat oven to 425°F. Spray a 9-inch pie plate with vegetable spray and line it with pie crust. Partially bake crust blind according to directions.

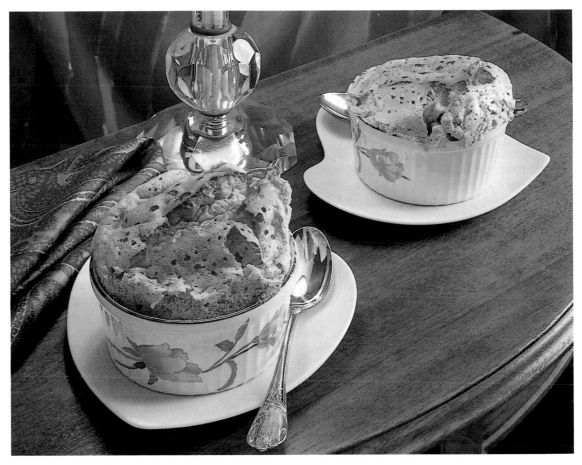

Light Coffee Soufflé (page 106)

Put blueberries into a large bowl. Halve tangerine sections and add blueberries. Toss with cornstarch and cinnamon. Add honey and toss again.

Fill prepared piecrust with mixture. Cover with foil but do not let it touch filling. Bake on middle shelf of oven until crust is golden and filling bubbly, about 45 minutes.

Remove foil and allow to cool. Serve warm or cold.

Makes 8 servings
(145 calories per serving)

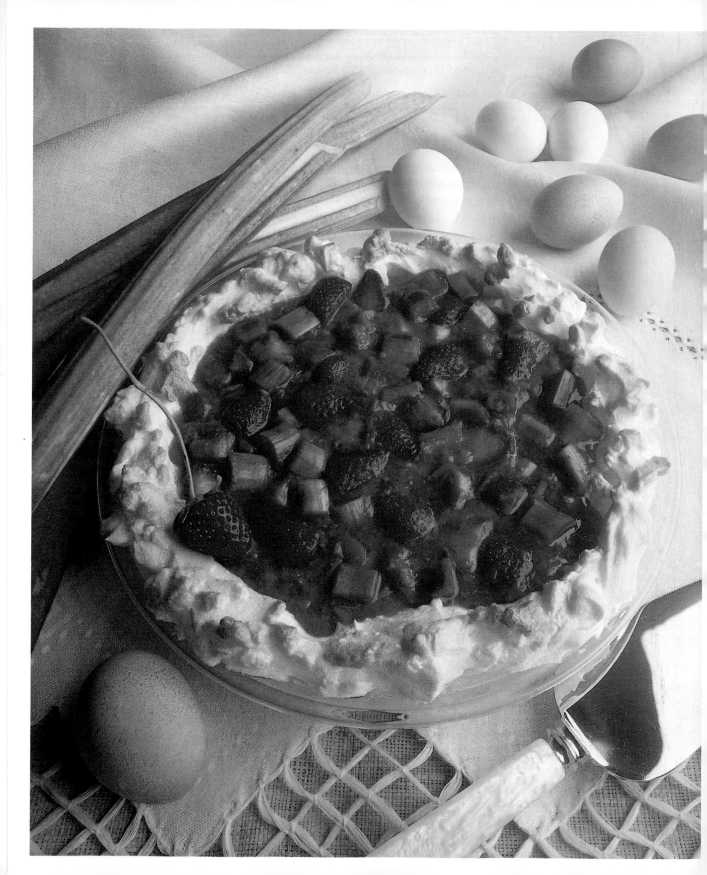

Peachy Raspberry Torte

This is a showy finish for a company meal.

4 egg whites, at room temperature
⅛ teaspoon cream of tartar
3 tablespoons honey
1 teaspoon vanilla extract
2 fresh peaches
1 cup fresh raspberries
1 cup Slim Pastry Cream
   (page 270)

Preheat oven to 275°F. Butter and lightly flour a large baking sheet. With a 7-inch saucepan cover, mark 2 circles on baking sheet.

In a large bowl, beat egg whites until foamy. Add cream of tartar. Gradually drizzle in honey and vanilla, beating until stiff peaks form. Divide between circles on baking sheet, spreading mixture to edges of circles. Bake on middle shelf of oven 40 to 45 minutes.

Cool meringues before removing from baking sheet. Just before serving, peel, pit, and chop peaches. In a medium-size bowl, mix them, along with raspberries, into pastry cream. Put half of the fruit mixture on the first meringue, spreading to edges. Place the second meringue on top and spread with remaining fruit mixture.

Makes 8 to 10 servings
(112 to 90 calories per serving)

Lime Chiffon Pie

1 recipe for Meringue Pie Shell
   (page 117)
1 envelope unflavored gelatin
3 tablespoons freshly squeezed
   lime juice
2 egg yolks
⅓ cup honey
1 teaspoon vanilla extract
½ cup evaporated skim milk, chilled
   natural green food coloring,
   optional
4 thin slices lime, halved, optional

Bake pie shell according to directions.

Sprinkle gelatin over lime juice and set aside for 5 minutes to soften.

In top of a double boiler, beat together egg yolks and honey. Beat in lime-gelatin mixture. Set over hot water and cook over low heat. Continue beating until gelatin dissolves, about 7 minutes. Remove from heat, and beat in vanilla. Allow to cool.

In a large, chilled bowl, beat evaporated skim milk until the consistency of whipped cream. Fold in lime mixture and green food coloring. Turn into pie shell and refrigerate until set.

Before serving, decorate with lime slices, if desired.

Makes 8 servings
(88 calories per serving)

Strawberry Rhubarb Pie with Meringue Crust (page 120)

Company Punch

7 cups pineapple juice
2 cups grapefruit juice
5 cups freshly squeezed orange
   juice
2 cups white grape juice
¼ cup honey, warmed

Mix all ingredients together. Chill and serve in a punch bowl over ice cubes.

Makes 32 servings
(80 calories per serving)

Papaya Baskets

2 very ripe papayas
1 cup quartered fresh strawberries,
   divided
¼ cup freshly squeezed orange juice,
   divided
¼ cup Delicious Diet Cream
   (page 119), divided

Halve papayas and scoop out seeds. Pile ¼ cup of the strawberries into each papaya half. Pour 1 tablespoon of the orange juice over each papaya half. Top each serving with 1 tablespoon of the diet cream.

Makes 4 servings
(84 calories per serving)

Applesauce Meringue

This loose, saucy pudding is a splendid dessert either warm or chilled.

2 eggs, separated
3 tablespoons honey, divided
½ cup part-skim ricotta cheese
1 teaspoon vanilla extract
1 teaspoon ground cinnamon
2 cups unsweetened Applesauce
   (page 90)
⅛ teaspoon cream of tartar

Preheat oven to 350°F. Spray a 1½-quart casserole with vegetable spray.

In a large bowl, beat egg yolks and 2 tablespoons of the honey until thick and light colored. Beat in ricotta, vanilla, and cinnamon. Fold in Applesauce and turn into prepared casserole. Bake on middle shelf of oven for 50 to 60 minutes.

Remove from oven and allow to cool slightly.

In a medium-size bowl, beat egg whites until foamy. Add cream of tartar and continue beating, drizzling in remaining honey, until stiff peaks form. Spread on top of pudding, sealing edges with beaten whites. Return to oven and bake until meringue is golden brown, 8 to 10 minutes.

Makes 8 servings
(81 calories per serving)

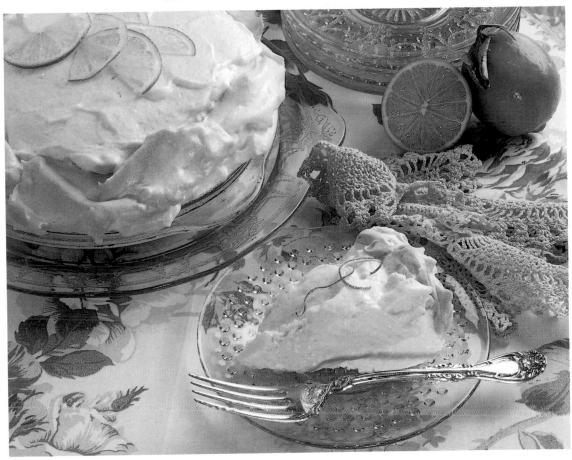

Lime Chiffon Pie (page 115)

Delicious Diet Cream

1 20-ounce can evaporated
    skim milk, chilled

1 tablespoon honey
1½ teaspoons vanilla extract

In a large, chilled bowl, beat evaporated skim milk until foamy. Add honey and vanilla and beat to the consistency of whipped cream. Use immediately.

Makes about 6 cups
(3 calories per tablespoon)

Papaya Fluff

1 **very ripe papaya**
⅓ **cup evaporated skim milk, chilled**
1 **tablespoon honey**
½ **teaspoon orange extract**

Peel, seed, and cut papaya into chunks. Puree in a food processor or blender.

In a medium-size bowl, beat evaporated skim milk until foamy. Add honey and orange extract and continue beating until stiff peaks form. Beat in papaya puree until blended.

Makes 4 servings
(63 calories per serving)

Strawberry Rhubarb Pie with Meringue Crust

1 **recipe for Meringue Pie Shell (page 117)**
2 **envelopes unflavored gelatin**
1½ **cups water, divided**
2¼ **cups chopped fresh rhubarb**
1½ **cups chopped fresh strawberries**
½ **cup honey**

Bake pie shell according to directions.

In a small bowl, sprinkle gelatin over ½ cup of the water. Set aside for 5 minutes to soften.

In a medium-size saucepan, combine rhubarb, strawberries, honey, and

remaining water. Bring to a boil over medium-high heat. Reduce heat and simmer for 5 minutes, stirring often. Add gelatin and stir until dissolved. Pour into a large bowl and refrigerate until thickened but not set.

Pour into pie shell and chill until set.

Makes 10 servings
(80 calories per serving)

Banana Strawberry Freeze

2 **cups halved fresh strawberries**
2 **large ripe bananas, chunked**
3 **tablespoons honey**
1 **cup skim milk**
1 **teaspoon vanilla extract**

Drop strawberries and bananas through feed tube of a food processor while machine is running and then add honey. Turn mixture into a large bowl. Mix in skim milk and vanilla.

Process mixture in an ice cream maker according to manufacturer's instructions, or place in freezer until partially frozen. Remove from freezer, beat to break down ice crystals, and then return to freezer. Repeat last procedure twice, spooning mixture into 2 1-quart containers the last time. Freeze until ready to serve.

Makes 8 servings
(82 calories per serving)

Carnation Cassata

12 Ladyfingers (page 108)
1½ cups unsweetened frozen rasp-
    berries, thawed
½ teaspoon rum extract
1 envelope unflavored gelatin
2 cups creamed cottage cheese
¼ cup honey, divided
½ cup evaporated skim milk,
    chilled
1 teaspoon vanilla extract

Line a 1½-quart casserole with plastic wrap. Arrange Ladyfingers in a single layer on top of plastic wrap.

Thoroughly drain raspberries, reserving juice in a small saucepan. Stir rum extract into reserved juice. Drizzle ¼ cup of the juice over Ladyfingers. Sprinkle gelatin over remaining juice and set aside to soften for 5 minutes.

In a large bowl, beat cottage cheese until fairly smooth. Add 3 tablespoons of the honey and beat until well blended.

Heat gelatin mixture over medium heat until gelatin dissolves. Remove from heat and beat into cheese mixture. Pour over Ladyfingers. Chill until set.

Turn dessert out onto a serving plate, carefully removing plastic wrap. Just before serving, beat evaporated skim milk in a small bowl until foamy. Drizzle in remaining honey and vanilla, and continue beating until milk is the consistency of whipped cream. Spread on cassata, top with raspberries, and serve.

Makes 10 servings
(145 calories per serving)

Strawberry Peach Pie

1 recipe for Coconut Crust
    (page 18)
3 cups fresh or unsweetened
    frozen whole strawberries
¼ cup honey
¼ cup freshly squeezed orange juice
3 tablespoons cornstarch
1 cup unsweetened frozen chunked
    peaches, thawed

Prepare Coconut Crust according to directions. Set aside to cool.

In a medium-size saucepan, combine strawberries and honey. In a jar with a tight-fitting lid, shake together orange juice and cornstarch. Add to strawberry mixture and heat, stirring constantly, until mixture thickens and becomes almost translucent. Set aside to cool.

When both piecrust and strawberries are cool, place peach chunks on bottom of piecrust. Spread strawberries on top and refrigerate until set.

Makes 10 servings
(113 calories per serving)

JUNE

Tips on Successful Dieting

FRUIT OF THE MONTH: **PEACHES**

DESSERT OF THE MONTH: **PRETTY PEACH LAYER CAKE**

DRINK OF THE MONTH: **ALMOND PEACH TREAT**

				1	2	3
				ENGLISH TEA CAKE	FROZEN PEACH BRANDY SUPREME	PUFFY APRICOT SOUFFLÉ
4	5	6	7	8	9	10
EASY GRAPE-NUTS CHERRY PUDDING	CREAMY FROZEN STRAWBERRY PIE	KISSEL	PRETTY PEACH LAYER CAKE ★	PAPAYA CUSTARD	FRUIT FONDUE	PEACHY BANANA CREPES
11	12	13	14	Father's Day 15	16	17
MELON RING WITH STRAWBERRIES	TWO-BERRY PIE	PEACH ALMOND ICE	RASPBERRY CHEESE PIE	BEST EVER BLUEBERRY PUFFS	LIGHT LEMON COOKIES	POLISH BERRY SOUP
18	19	20	21	22	23	24
PERFECT PLUM PIE	NECTARINE CUPS	BLUEBERRY RAISIN CAKE	FROZEN PEACH SOUFFLÉ	EASY STRAWBERRY RICE PUDDING	ORIENTAL APRICOT PIE	CHERRY ORANGE DELIGHT
25	26	27	28	29	30	
ONE SUCCULENT RIPE PEACH	STRAWBERRY SHELLS WITH RASPBERRY SAUCE	PAPAYA MILK SHAKE	PINEAPPLE SURPRISE	MELLOW MELON COMPOTE	PEACHY ALMOND CAKE	

Strawberry Shells with Raspberry Sauce (page 134)

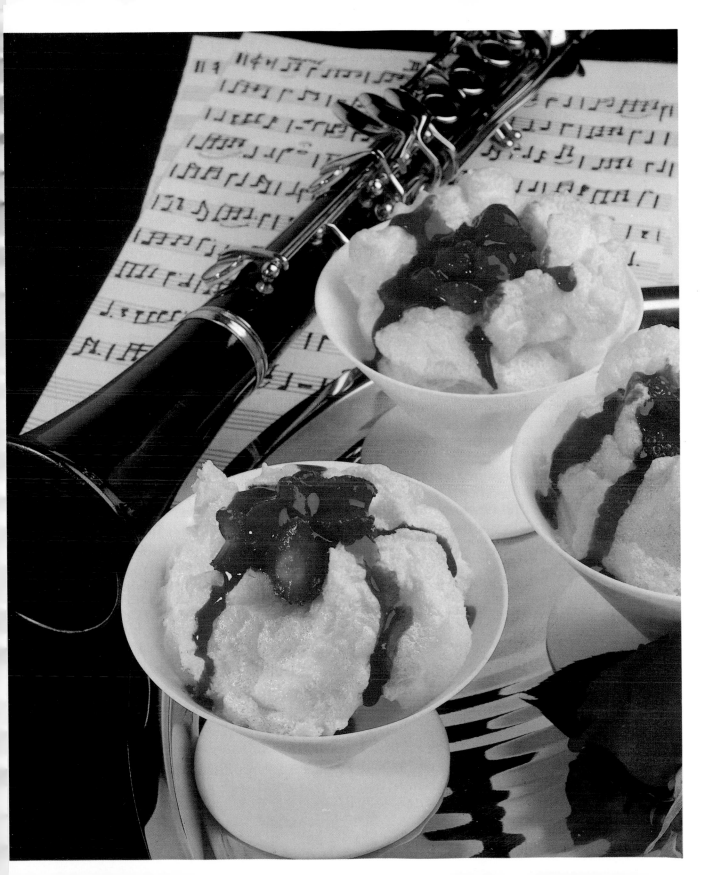

English Tea Cake

This light and tasty cake is frequently served in England at tea time.

> 3 eggs
> ⅓ cup honey
> 1 teaspoon vanilla extract
> 1 teaspoon almond extract
> ⅔ cup whole wheat pastry flour
> ⅔ cup unbleached white flour
> 1 teaspoon baking powder
> 2 tablespoons red currant jelly
> 2 teaspoons red grape juice

Preheat oven to 350°F. Spray bottom of an 8 × 8-inch pan with vegetable spray. Line bottom with parchment paper.

In a large bowl, beat together eggs, honey, and extracts until very thick, at least 7 minutes.

In a medium-size bowl, sift together whole wheat pastry flour, unbleached white flour, and baking powder, stirring with a wire whisk to blend. Fold into beaten eggs and turn into prepared pan, carefully smoothing top. Bake on middle shelf of oven for 20 minutes.

Cool 10 minutes in pan. Run knife around edges of pan and turn cake out onto a wire rack. Remove parchment paper and allow to cool completely.

In a small saucepan, melt jelly with grape juice. Set aside to cool until slightly thickened, about 5 minutes. Brush on top of cake.

Makes 24 tea squares
(52 calories per square)

Frozen Peach Brandy Supreme

The small amount of half-and-half used in this recipe gives it a deceptively creamy texture.

> 16 ounces unsweetened frozen
>   peaches, thawed
> ¼ cup apricot preserves
> 1 teaspoon brandy extract
> 2 teaspoons vanilla extract
> 2 teaspoons almond extract
> 1 tablespoon honey
> 1½ cups skim milk
> ½ cup half-and-half

In a food processor, puree peaches and preserves. Add extracts and process just to blend. Mix together honey, skim milk, and half-and-half in a large bowl. Add peach mixture and stir to mix.

Process mixture in an ice cream maker according to manufacturer's instructions, or turn mixture into a large, square pan and freeze until thickened but not frozen. Remove from freezer, beat to break down ice crystals, and then return to freezer. Repeat this procedure twice, packing ice milk into 2 1-quart containers the last time. Freeze until ready to serve.

Makes 8 servings
(93 calories per serving)

Puffy Apricot Soufflé

4 egg whites
¼ teaspoon cream of tartar
3 tablespoons honey
1 teaspoon vanilla extract
1 cup apricot puree (6 to 7 fresh
    apricots, peeled and pureed in
    a food processor)

Preheat oven to 300°F. Spray a 2-quart casserole with vegetable spray.

In a large bowl, beat egg whites until foamy. Add cream of tartar and continue beating, drizzling in honey and vanilla, until stiff peaks form. Fold in puree and turn into prepared casserole. Set casserole in a pan of warm water and bake on middle shelf of oven until puffy and browned, about 30 minutes. Serve immediately.

Makes 6 servings
(60 calories per serving)

Easy Grape-Nuts Cherry Pudding

2 tablespoons quick-cooking
    tapioca
2 tablespoons honey
1 egg yolk
2 cups skim milk
½ teaspoon almond extract
1 cup pitted and chopped fresh
    sweet cherries, divided
4 teaspoons grape-nuts cereal,
    divided
4 fresh sweet cherries, pitted

In a medium-size saucepan, mix together tapioca, honey, egg yolk, and skim milk. Set aside for 5 minutes for tapioca to soften.

Bring mixture to a boil and cook over medium heat for 6 to 8 minutes, stirring constantly. Remove from heat and stir in extract. Cool 20 to 30 minutes.

Divide half the pudding among 4 dessert dishes. Sprinkle ¼ cup of the chopped cherries over each serving. Divide remaining pudding among the 4 dishes, spreading over cherries. Sprinkle 1 teaspoon of the grape-nuts over each portion, top with a whole cherry, and serve.

Makes 4 servings
(134 calories per serving)

★ Pretty Peach Layer Cake

½ cup whole wheat pastry flour
½ cup unbleached white flour
1 teaspoon baking powder
2 eggs
⅓ cup plus 1 tablespoon honey
4 teaspoons freshly squeezed
    lemon juice, divided
¼ cup skim milk
4 fresh peaches
1 tablespoon honey
1 cup Delicious Diet Cream
    (page 119)

Preheat oven to 350°F.

Sift together whole wheat pastry flour, unbleached white flour, and baking powder into a small bowl. Whisk to blend.

In a large bowl, beat eggs until thick and light, about 7 minutes. Drizzle in ⅓ cup of the honey and 2 teaspoons of the lemon juice, beating for another minute.

In a small saucepan, scald skim milk.

Sift flour mixture into egg mixture gradually, folding in. Mix in hot milk quickly. Turn into 2 8-inch layer cake pans with nonstick surfaces. Bake on middle shelf of oven until cakes spring back when pressed lightly, 15 to 20 minutes.

Cool in pans inverted on wire racks.

In a small bowl, combine remaining lemon juice and remaining honey.

Peel, pit, and slice peaches. Toss with juice and honey. Put half of peaches on 1 cake layer. Top with other layer. Spread diet cream on top and arrange remaining peaches on cream.

Makes 16 servings
(87 calories per serving)

Fruit Fondue

¾ cup plain low-fat yogurt
½ cup Ruby Raspberry Sauce
    (page 139)
8 fresh strawberries
1 fresh peach
1 medium-size kiwi fruit
16 seedless green grapes

In a small bowl, combine yogurt and raspberry sauce. Chill. Before serving stir to mix.

Cut strawberries into halves. Peel, pit, and cut peach into 16 pieces. Peel and cut kiwi into eight slices, then halve slices.

Serve dip in a small bowl in the center of a plate. Surround with fruit pieces and grapes.

Makes 8 servings
(36 calories per serving)

Creamy Frozen Strawberry Pie

1 recipe for Mini Piecrust
    (page 113)
1 envelope unflavored gelatin
½ cup water
3 tablespoons honey, divided
1½ cups unsweetened frozen straw-
    berries, thawed
¾ cup evaporated skim milk,
    chilled
1 teaspoon vanilla extract

Bake piecrust according to directions. Cool thoroughly.

In a small saucepan, sprinkle gelatin over water. Set aside for 5 minutes to soften. Heat over medium heat, stirring constantly, until gelatin dissolves. Stir in 1 tablespoon of the honey.

In a food processor, puree strawberries. Stir together gelatin mixture and pureed strawberries in a medium-size bowl. Chill until thickened but not set, about 30 minutes.

In a large bowl, beat evaporated skim milk until foamy. Add vanilla and remaining honey and beat until the consistency of whipped cream. Beat in strawberry mixture and turn into cooled pie shell. Freeze until ready to serve.

Makes 8 servings
(114 calories per serving)

Peachy Banana Crepes

1 large ripe banana
¼ cup Peach Sauce (page 132)
½ teaspoon vanilla extract
¼ teaspoon freshly squeezed lemon juice
4 warm Delicious Diet Crepes (page 33)
¼ cup plain low-fat yogurt, divided
4 fresh strawberries, optional

In a medium-size bowl, mash banana with Peach Sauce, vanilla extract, and lemon juice. Spread on crepes and roll up. Top each crepe with 1 tablespoon yogurt and a strawberry, if desired.

Makes 4 servings
(93 calories per serving)

Melon Ring with Strawberries

2 envelopes unflavored gelatin
⅔ cup boiling water
1¾ cup white grape juice
2 tablespoons freshly squeezed lemon juice
2 cups fresh cantaloupe balls
1 pint fresh strawberries
1 cup Mock Whipped Cream (page 10), optional

Dissolve gelatin in boiling water. Transfer to a medium-size bowl. Add grape juice and lemon juice, mixing well. Rinse a 4-cup ring mold in cold water. Distribute melon balls evenly inside mold. Pour gelatin mixture over melon balls and chill until set.

Unmold gelatin ring by running a knife around edges and then inverting it onto a plate, putting a tea towel wrung out in hot water on top of mold.

Fill center of unmolded gelatin ring with strawberries and pipe Mock Whipped Cream around bottom edge, if desired.

Makes 8 servings
(84 calories per serving)

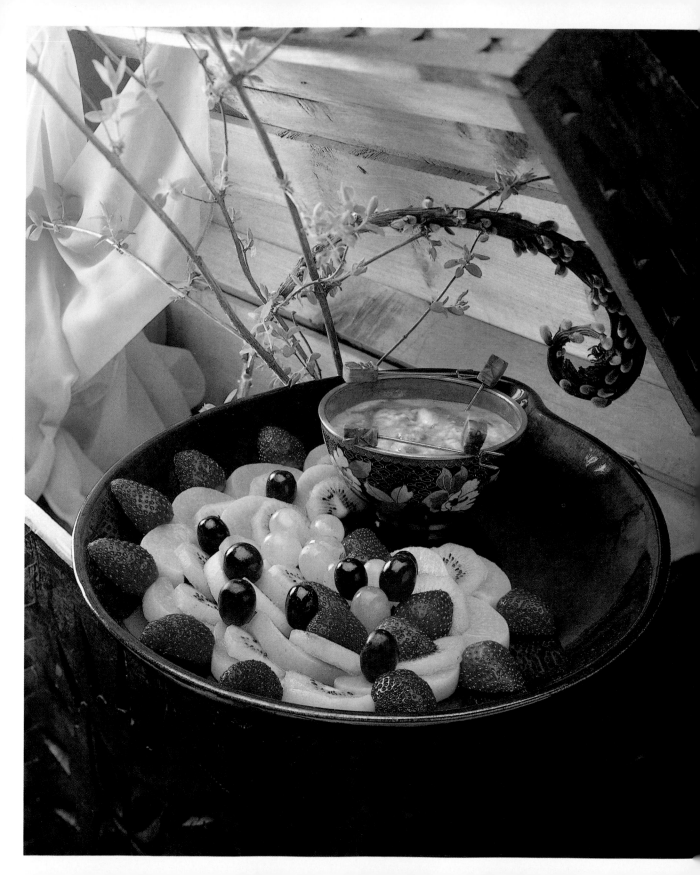

Two-Berry Pie

*This one-crust pie should be completely
cooled before it's sliced or it will be runny.*

- 2 cups fresh blueberries
- 2 cups fresh raspberries
- ½ cup water
- 3 tablespoons quick-cooking
  tapioca
- ⅓ cup honey
- 1 teaspoon almond extract
- 1 recipe for Mini Piecrust
  (page 113)

Preheat oven to 450°F. Spray a 9-inch
pie plate with vegetable spray.

In a medium-size bowl, toss berries
together.

In a small bowl, mix water and tapioca together and set aside for 5 minutes
for tapioca to soften. Stir in honey and
extract. Mix into berries well and turn
into prepared pie plate, mounding slightly
higher in center.

Roll out piecrust according to directions and place on top of fruit, crimping
around edge with a fork. Cut generous
vents in crust and bake on middle shelf
of oven for 10 minutes. Reduce heat to
350°F and continue to bake until crust
is lightly browned, about 30 minutes.

Makes 8 servings
(152 calories per serving)

Easy Strawberry Rice Pudding

- 2½ cups water
- 1 cup brown rice
- 2 eggs
- 2 tablespoons honey
- 1½ cups skim milk
- 1 teaspoon vanilla extract
- ½ teaspoon strawberry extract
- 1 cup fresh strawberries, quartered

In a large saucepan, heat water and
rice to boiling. Reduce heat, cover, and
simmer until rice is soft, about 40 to
45 minutes.

In a medium-size bowl, beat eggs
and honey. Stir in skim milk. Mix into
rice and continue cooking, stirring
constantly, until mixture thickens, about
15 minutes.

Remove from heat. Stir in extracts
and strawberries.

Makes 10 servings
(115 calories per serving)

Fruit Fondue (page 128)

Cherry Orange Delight

1 envelope unflavored gelatin
1 cup water
3 ounces unsweetened frozen
   orange juice concentrate
1 tablespoon honey
1½ cups unsweetened frozen
   cherries

In a small saucepan, sprinkle gelatin over water. Set aside to soften for 5 minutes. Heat over medium heat, stirring constantly, until gelatin dissolves. Pour into a blender and process with remaining ingredients until liquified. Pour into dessert dishes and chill until set.

Makes 5 servings
(84 calories per serving)

Strawberry Shells with Raspberry Sauce

1 recipe for Meringue Shells
   (page 84)
2 cups coarsely chopped fresh
   strawberries, divided
¾ cup Ruby Raspberry Sauce
   (page 139), divided

Bake Meringue Shells according to directions.

Spoon ⅓ cup of the strawberries into each Meringue Shell. Top with 2 tablespoons of the raspberry sauce and serve immediately.

Makes 6 servings
(50 calories per serving)

Blueberry Grape Sauce

A tablespoon of this sauce will add zip to a serving of ice milk, a piece of cake, a crepe, or a dish of pudding.

1½ cups unsweetened frozen
   blueberries, thawed
½ cup red grape juice

2 teaspoons cornstarch
½ cup water
1 tablespoon honey

In a medium-size saucepan, mix together blueberries and grape juice. Dissolve cornstarch in water and add to blueberries. Stir in honey. Cook over medium heat, stirring constantly, until mixture bubbles and thickens.

Remove from heat.
Serve warm.

Makes about 2 cups
(10 calories per tablespoon)

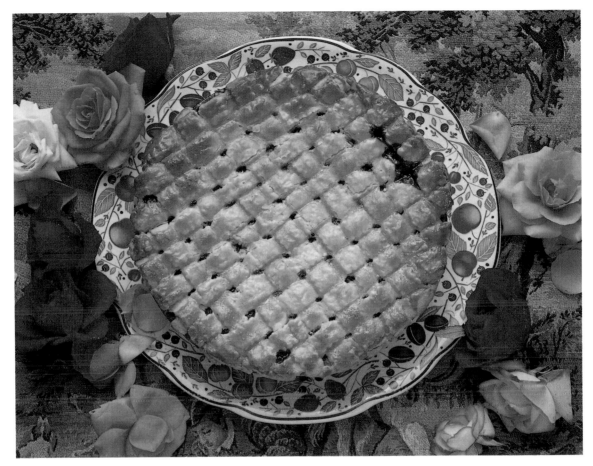

Two-Berry Pie (page 131)

Papaya Custard

1 papaya
1 cup Slim Pastry Cream (page 270)

Peel, seed, and dice papaya.

In a medium-size bowl, mix fruit with pastry cream. Divide among 4 dessert glasses. Chill before serving.

Makes 4 servings
(95 calories per serving)

Papaya Milk Shake

2 cups skim milk
¾ cup chopped papaya pulp
2 tablespoons honey

In a food processor, blend all ingredients until very smooth. Serve immediately.

Makes 4 servings
(86 calories per serving)

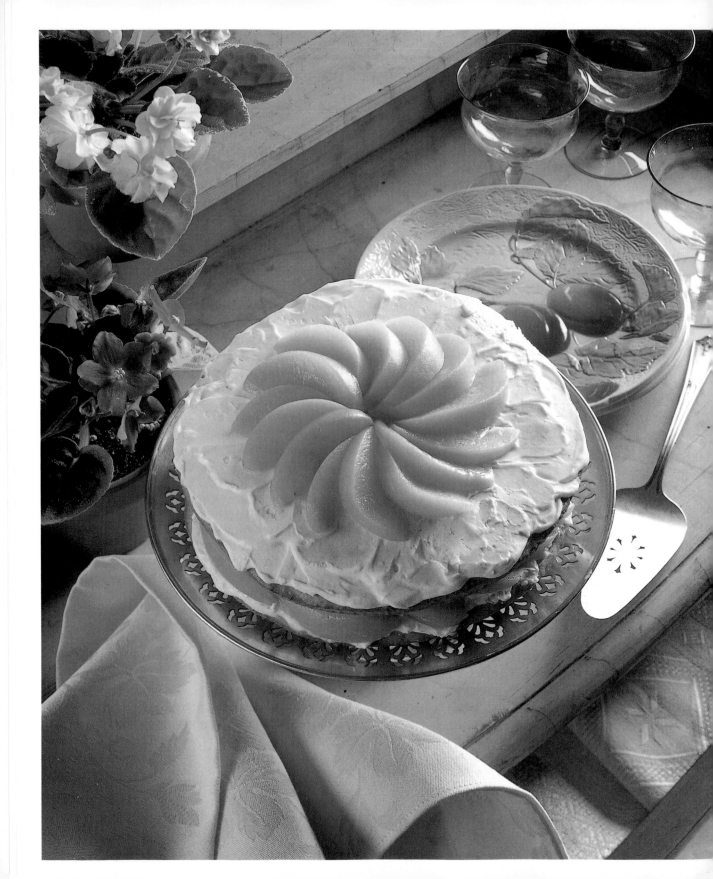

Kissel

Currants are traditional in Kissel, but the remaining fruit is optional.

1 tablespoon cornstarch
½ cup water
2 tablespoons honey
½ cup red currants
½ cup peeled, pitted, chopped fresh apricots
½ cup fresh blueberries
1 cup fresh raspberries

In a jar with a tight-fitting lid, shake together cornstarch and water. Pour into a medium-size saucepan. Stir in honey. Add currants and apricots and heat over medium heat, stirring constantly, until mixture thickens and fruit is soft. Add blueberries and cook 30 seconds. Stir in raspberries and cook an additional 30 seconds. Allow to cool before serving.

Makes 4 servings
(123 calories per serving)

Frozen Peach Soufflé

3 fresh peaches, peeled, pitted, and quartered
½ cup honey
2 eggs, separated
1 teaspoon vanilla extract
⅛ teaspoon cream of tartar

In a food processor, puree peaches and honey. Pour into top of a double boiler. Beat egg yolks in a small bowl and stir into peach mixture. Cook over simmering, but not boiling, water for 10 minutes, stirring constantly. Remove from heat and set aside to cool.

In a medium-size bowl, beat egg whites until foamy, add cream of tartar, and continue beating until stiff peaks form. Fold beaten egg whites into cooled peach mixture. Turn into a 4-cup mold. Cover and freeze.

Makes 6 servings
(132 calories per serving)

Pretty Peach Layer Cake (page 128)

Almond Peach Treat

1 cup peeled, very ripe peach
   chunks
1 cup skim milk
1 teaspoon honey
¼ teaspoon almond extract
½ teaspoon vanilla extract

Puree peach chunks in a blender. Add remaining ingredients. Process and serve immediately.

Makes 3 servings
(60 calories per serving)

Peachy Almond Cake

2 eggs
½ cup honey
⅓ cup vegetable oil
1 teaspoon almond extract
¾ cup whole wheat pastry flour
¾ cup unbleached white flour
2 teaspoons baking powder
1½ teaspoons ground cinnamon
2 fresh peaches, peeled, pitted,
   and chopped

Preheat oven to 325°F. Spray an 8 × 8-inch pan with vegetable spray.

In a large bowl, beat together eggs, honey, oil, and almond extract.

In a medium-size bowl, sift together whole wheat pastry flour, unbleached white flour, baking powder, and cinnamon. Add to beaten ingredients. Mix together thoroughly. Stir peaches into batter and turn into prepared pan. Bake on middle shelf of oven until a cake tester inserted into center comes out clean, about 35 minutes.

Makes 12 servings
(172 calories per serving)

Nectarine Cups

¼ cup nonfat dry milk
¼ cup cold water
1½ teaspoons freshly squeezed
    lemon juice
1 tablespoon honey
3 fresh nectarines, peeled, pitted,
    and halved
¾ cup Strawberry Sauce (page 253),
    divided

In a small bowl, mix nonfat dry milk and water together. Add lemon juice and beat until light and fluffy. Beat in honey.

Put each nectarine half in a sherbet glass and spoon whipped lemon mixture over them. Top with Strawberry Sauce. Serve immediately.

Makes 6 servings
(104 calories per serving)

JULY

Calorie-Controlled Cakes

FRUIT OF THE MONTH: **RASPBERRIES**
DESSERT OF THE MONTH: **FRESH RASPBERRY CREAM PIE**
DRINK OF THE MONTH: **SPARKLING PUNCH**

				1 LIGHT RHUBARB CREPES	2 FRENCH VANILLA CHERRY ICE MILK	3 PEACHY BLUEBERRY FLUFF
Independence Day 4 FOURTH OF JULY SPECTACULAR	5 MELON SOUP	6 APRICOT RAISIN PIE	7 CHEESECAKE FRAMBOISE	8 FAUX CHERRIES JUBILEE	9 PLUM ORANGE ICE	10 SUPER FRUIT KABOBS
11 ALMOND BAVARIAN CREAM WITH KIWI FRUITS	12 CHERRY TORTE	13 PEACH BARS	14 FRESH RASPBERRY CREAM PIE ★	15 LIGHT CAROB MOUSSE	16 POACHED GINGER PEACHES IN CUSTARD	17 GRAPE BANANA GELATIN LAYERS
18 MINI CAKE ROLLS	19 ORANGE LEMON FLUFF	20 HONEYDEW SHERBET	21 SHILEM TOUFU	22 ORANGE PINEAPPLE SHAKE	23 PEACH YOGURT WHIP	24 ½ CUP FRESH RASPBERRIES WITH 2 TABLESPOONS DELICIOUS DIET CREAM
25 BEAUTIFUL BLACKBERRY PIE	26 ALMOND-FLAVORED PECAN COOKIES	27 CAROB TRUFFLES	28 RASPBERRY RUM SHERBET	29 CAROB-DIPPED TANGERINES	30 THREE-MELON COMPOTE	31 RASPBERRY COCONUT PIE

144

Three-Melon Compote (page 166)

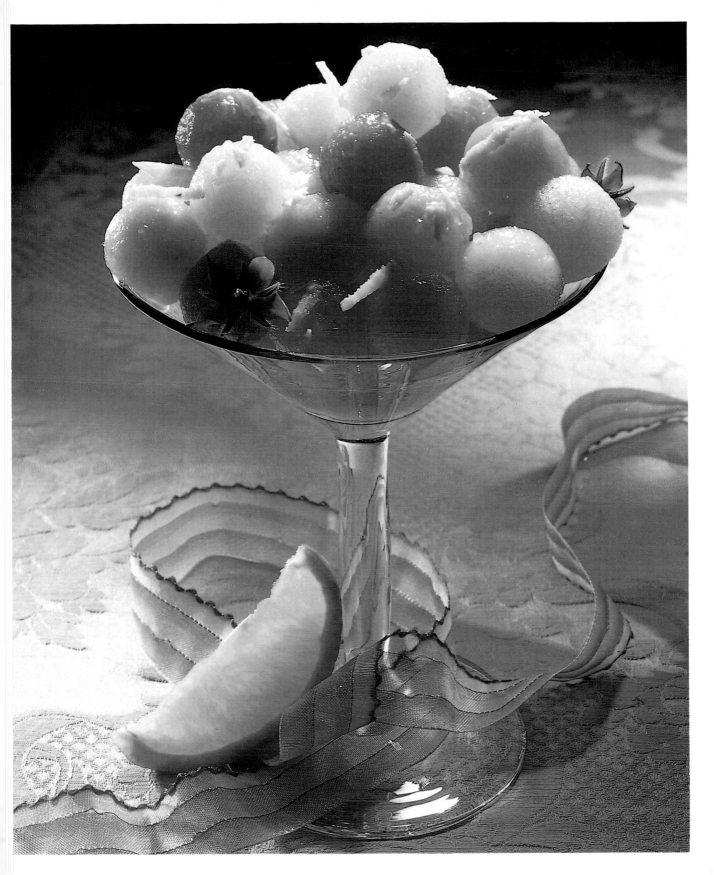

Peachy Blueberry Fluff

¾ cup evaporated skim milk,
   chilled
1 tablespoon honey
½ teaspoon vanilla extract
1 large ripe peach, peeled, pitted,
   and pureed
½ cup fresh blueberries

In a medium-size bowl, beat together skim milk, honey, and vanilla to the consistency of whipped cream. Fold in peach puree and blueberries and serve immediately.

Makes 2 servings
(161 calories per serving)

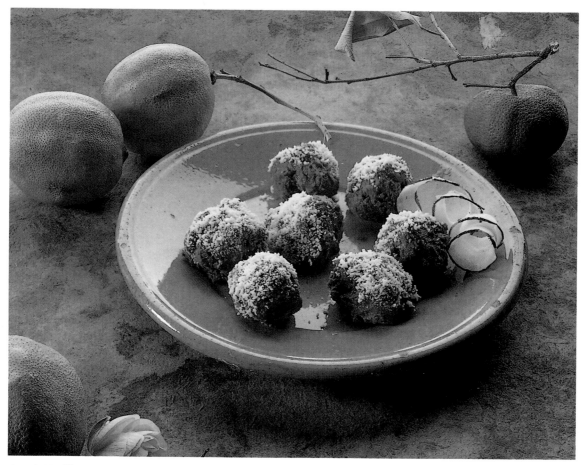

Carob Truffles (page 167)

Peach Bars

These firm bars are very filling.

 1 cup whole wheat pastry flour
 1 cup unbleached white flour
1½ teaspoons baking powder
1½ teaspoons ground cinnamon
 ¼ teaspoon ground nutmeg
 ¼ cup butter, softened
 ¼ cup part-skim ricotta cheese
 ½ cup honey
 2 eggs
 1 4½-ounce jar strained peaches

Preheat oven to 350°F. Spray a 9 × 13-inch pan with vegetable spray.

Sift together whole wheat pastry flour, unbleached white flour, baking powder, cinnamon, and nutmeg into a medium-size bowl.

In a large bowl, beat butter and cheese together until smooth. Beat in honey, eggs, and peaches. Gradually mix in flour. Turn batter into prepared pan, spreading evenly. Bake on middle shelf of oven for 35 to 40 minutes.

Cool in pan, then cut into 36 bars.

Makes 36 bars
(65 calories per bar)

Cherry Torte

 1 recipe for Pretty Peach Layer
   Cake (page 128)
 1 envelope unflavored gelatin
 ½ cup water
 1 tablespoon honey
 ½ cup freshly squeezed orange
   juice
1½ cups pitted fresh sweet cherries

Bake cake according to directions.

In a small saucepan, sprinkle gelatin over water. Set aside to soften for 5 minutes. Heat, stirring constantly, until gelatin dissolves. Stir in honey, then orange juice. Chill until quite thick but not set, 30 to 40 minutes.

Wrap and freeze 1 layer of the cake for future use. Place the second layer on a serving plate. Arrange cherries on top of cake. Spoon gelatin mixture evenly over cherries and cake, spreading to edges. It's all right for gelatin to run down sides of cake. Chill until set.

Makes 12 servings
(66 calories per serving)

Variation: To make a Strawberry Torte, substitute 1½ cups sliced fresh strawberries for the cherries and decorate center with a few whole berries. The number of calories per serving will be slightly less.

Mini Cake Rolls

1 recipe for Jelly Roll Cake
    (page 54)
¾ cup Ruby Raspberry Sauce
    (page 139)
¾ cup Tangy Lemon Filling
    (page 244)
¼ cup Coconut Sugar (page 66)

Bake Jelly Roll Cake according to directions.

Cut cake in half crosswise. Spread half of the cake with raspberry sauce and the second half with lemon filling. Cut each piece in half crosswise. Cut pieces into thirds. Roll up, jelly roll fashion, over filling, starting from short side. Cut jelly rolls into halves, making 2 rolls from each piece. Roll in Coconut Sugar.

Makes 24 mini rolls
(60 calories per roll)

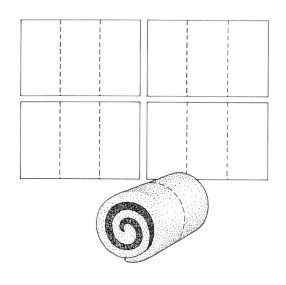

Orange Lemon Fluff

A cool treat for a hot day!

2 teaspoons unflavored gelatin
¼ cup water
2 eggs, separated
2 tablespoons honey
3 tablespoons freshly squeezed
    orange juice
1 tablespoon freshly squeezed
    lemon juice
2 egg whites
⅛ teaspoon cream of tartar
4 fresh orange sections, optional
4 mint leaves, optional

In a small saucepan, sprinkle gelatin over water. Set aside to soften for about 5 minutes, then heat over low heat, stirring constantly, until gelatin dissolves. Remove from heat.

In a small bowl, beat together egg yolks and honey. Pour a little gelatin mixture into beaten yolks, whisking constantly. Return to gelatin in saucepan, whisking well, and cook over low heat until mixture thickens slightly, about 8 minutes. Stir in orange juice and lemon juice. Pour into a small bowl and refrigerate until thickened but not set.

In a medium-size bowl, beat egg whites until foamy. Add cream of tartar and continue beating until stiff but not dry. Fold in orange-lemon mixture and divide among 4 dessert dishes. Chill until set.

If you wish, decorate each dish with an orange section and a mint leaf.

Makes 4 servings
(101 calories per serving)

Poached Ginger Peaches in Custard

4 cups water
½ cup honey
½ cup maple syrup
1 tablespoon freshly squeezed lemon juice
1 teaspoon ground cinnamon
1 teaspoon ground ginger
4 large, firm peaches
1½ cups Slim Pastry Cream (page 270)

In a medium-size saucepan, combine water, honey, maple syrup, lemon juice, cinnamon, and ginger. Bring to a boil. Reduce heat.

Halve, peel, and pit peaches. Set in poaching liquid and poach (water should be barely moving) until soft, about 10 minutes. Remove from liquid with a slotted spoon, allowing spices to cling to fruit. Place on a plate in a single layer to cool.

Whisk pastry cream briskly to loosen it. Spoon over peaches.

Makes 8 servings
(199 calories per serving)

Faux Cherries Jubilee

1 teaspoon cornstarch
¼ cup white grape juice
1 cup unsweetened frozen cherries, thawed
¼ teaspoon brandy extract
2 cups Vanilla Ice Milk (page 79)

In a small saucepan, dissolve cornstarch in grape juice. Add cherries and cook over medium heat, stirring constantly, until sauce thickens and turns red. Remove from heat and stir in brandy extract.

Divide ice milk among 4 dessert glasses. Divide sauce among glasses, spooning it over ice milk. Serve immediately.

Makes 4 servings
(186 calories per serving)

Honeydew Sherbet

1 large, ripe honeydew melon
¼ cup plus 2 tablespoons honey, divided
1½ cups evaporated skim milk, chilled

Peel, seed, and chunk melon. In a food processor, puree melon chunks. Add ¼ cup of the honey and process just to mix. Turn into a large saucepan and cook over medium heat, stirring constantly, for 5 minutes. Allow to cool.

In a large bowl, beat evaporated skim milk until soft peaks form. Drizzle in remaining honey, continuing to beat just until blended. Fold in cooled melon mixture.

Process mixture in an ice cream maker according to manufacturer's instructions, or turn mixture into a large shallow bowl or pan, cover, and freeze until mushy but not frozen. Remove from freezer, beat to break down ice crystals, and then return to freezer. Repeat this procedure twice, spooning mixture into a container the last time. Freeze until ready to serve.

Makes about 8 servings
(168 calories per serving)

Shilem Toufu (Almond Jelly)

2 envelopes unflavored gelatin
¾ cup water
3 cups skim milk
⅓ cup honey
1 teaspoon vanilla extract
1 teaspoon almond extract
1½ cups Peach Sauce (page 132), divided

In a medium-size saucepan, sprinkle gelatin over water. Set aside for 5 minutes to soften. Add skim milk and honey and heat over medium heat until gelatin dissolves, stirring constantly. Remove from heat and stir in extracts.

Allow to cool slightly, then divide among 6 dessert glasses. Chill until set.

At serving time spread ¼ cup of the Peach Sauce over each jelly.

Makes 6 servings
(148 calories per serving)

Cheesecake Framboise (page 152)

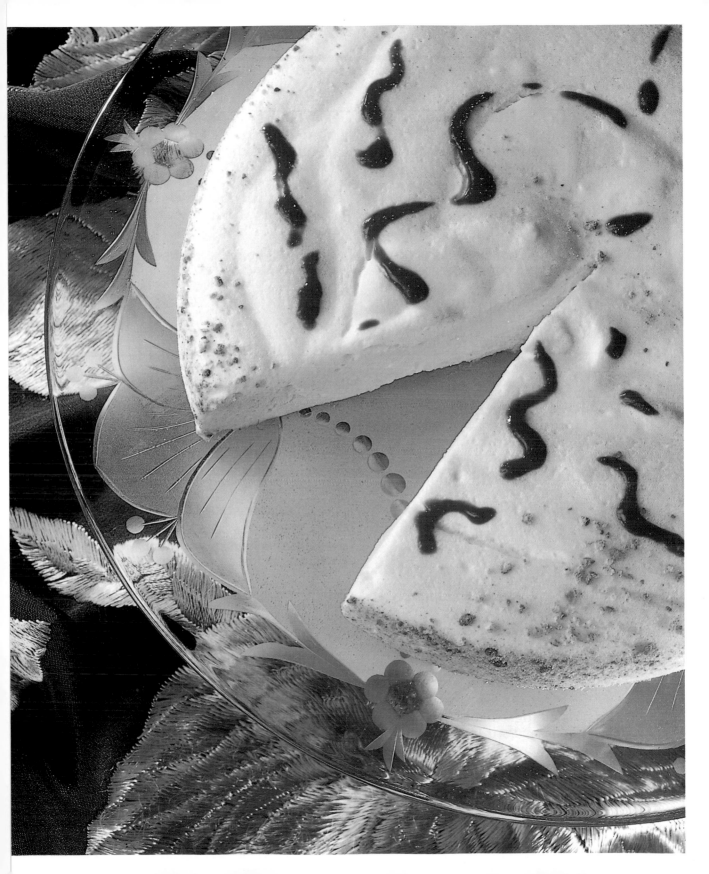

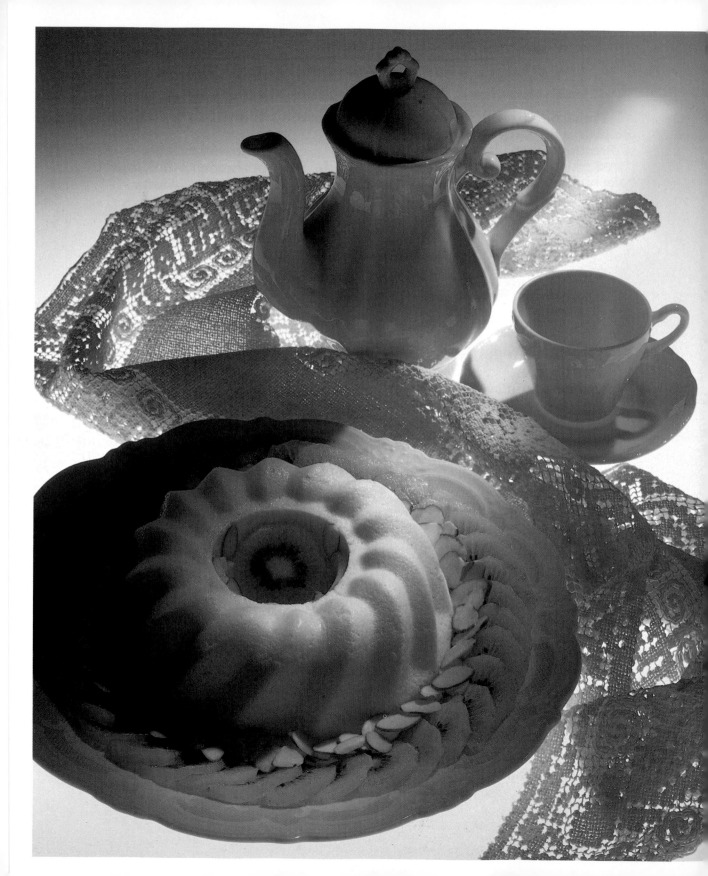

Grape Banana Gelatin Layers

1 envelope unflavored gelatin
1¼ cups cold water
1 6-ounce can unsweetened
   frozen grape juice concentrate
1 large, ripe banana

In a medium-size saucepan, sprinkle gelatin over water. Set aside for 5 minutes to soften. Heat until gelatin dissolves, stirring constantly. Remove from heat and stir in concentrate. Put in refrigerator until thickened but not set, 1 to 1½ hours.

Spoon a layer of gelatin mixture into each of 6 dessert glasses. Thinly slice banana. Make a banana layer on top of each gelatin layer. Continue to layer, ending with gelatin, until all ingredients are used. Chill until set.

Makes 6 servings
(78 calories per serving)

Raspberry Rum Sherbet

1 20-ounce package unsweetened
   frozen raspberries, thawed
2 eggs
½ cup honey
2 teaspoons freshly squeezed
   lemon juice
1½ cups skim milk
2 teaspoons rum extract

In a food processor, puree raspberries. Strain and discard seeds. (If you don't mind seeds, you don't have to strain puree.)

In a large bowl, beat eggs and honey until fluffy. Mix in raspberry puree, lemon juice, skim milk, and rum extract.

Process mixture in an ice cream maker according to manufacturer's directions, or turn mixture into a large shallow pan, cover, and freeze until thickened but not frozen. Remove from freezer, beat to break down ice crystals, and then return to freezer. Repeat this procedure twice, turning sherbet into 2 1-quart containers before returning to freezer the last time. Freeze until ready to serve.

Makes 8 servings
(171 calories per serving)

Almond Bavarian Cream with Kiwi Fruits (page 156)

Carob-Dipped Tangerines

2 tablespoons carob chips
1 tablespoon butter
16 tangerine sections
¼ cup Coconut Sugar (page 66)

In the top of a double boiler set over hot water, melt together carob chips and butter. Dip both ends of tangerine sections into melted carob, then dip them in Coconut Sugar. Place onto a baking sheet lined with waxed paper and refrigerate until carob is hardened.

Serve 2 sections to each person.

Makes 8 servings
(45 calories per serving)

Three-Melon Compote

½ large cantaloupe
½ large honeydew
¼ watermelon
¼ cup unsweetened flaked coconut
½ cup freshly squeezed orange juice

With a melon baller, make melon balls from cantaloupe, honeydew, and watermelon, removing watermelon seeds. Toss melon balls in a glass bowl with coconut and orange juice. Cover and chill.

Toss again before serving.

Makes 8 servings
(45 calories per serving)

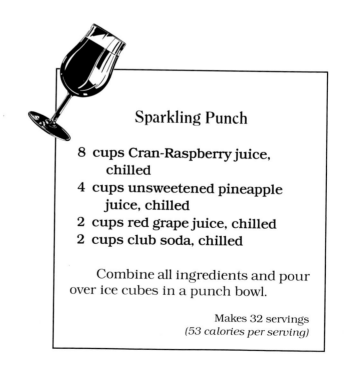

Sparkling Punch

8 cups Cran-Raspberry juice, chilled
4 cups unsweetened pineapple juice, chilled
2 cups red grape juice, chilled
2 cups club soda, chilled

Combine all ingredients and pour over ice cubes in a punch bowl.

Makes 32 servings
(53 calories per serving)

Raspberry Coconut Pie

1 recipe for Skinny Piecrust
  (page 6)
2 tablespoons cornstarch, divided
2 cups skim milk, divided
2 envelopes unflavored gelatin,
  divided
2 tablespoons honey, divided
1 teaspoon rum extract
½ cup unsweetened flaked coconut
1 20-ounce package unsweetened
  frozen raspberries, thawed

Line a 9-inch pie plate with pastry and bake according to directions.

In a medium-size saucepan, dissolve 1 tablespoon of the cornstarch in 1 cup of the skim milk. Sprinkle 1 envelope of the gelatin over milk and set aside to soften for 5 minutes. Add 1 tablespoon of the honey and heat over medium heat, stirring constantly, until mixture thickens and gelatin dissolves. Stir in rum extract, remaining milk, and coconut. Pour into prepared pie plate and chill until set, about 2 hours.

Drain raspberries, reserving juice in small saucepan. Place raspberries into a medium-size bowl. Stir into reserved juice remaining cornstarch and remaining honey. Sprinkle remaining gelatin over top. Set aside to soften for 5 minutes. Heat over medium heat, stirring constantly, until mixture thickens and gelatin dissolves. Remove from heat and stir into raspberries. Spread on top of coconut mixture and chill until set, preferably overnight.

Makes 8 servings
(151 calories per serving)

Carob Truffles

1 cup part-skim ricotta cheese
¼ cup honey
1 teaspoon vanilla extract
½ cup Coconut Sugar (page 66),
  divided
¼ cup carob chips
2 tablespoons butter

In a medium-size bowl, beat together ricotta, honey, vanilla, and ¼ cup Coconut Sugar until smooth.

In the top of a double boiler set over hot water, melt together carob chips and butter. Beat into cheese mixture and chill until easy to handle. Roll into 1-inch balls between palms of hands. Roll each ball in remaining Coconut Sugar, place on a baking sheet lined with waxed paper, and refrigerate.

Makes 3 dozen truffles
(27 calories per truffle)

AUGUST

Make Your Diet Desserts Ahead

FRUIT OF THE MONTH: **PLUMS**

DESSERT OF THE MONTH: **VANILLA PLUM PIE**

DRINK OF THE MONTH: **MINTED LEMONADE**

				1	2	3
				PEACH MELBA CREPE CUPS	GRAPE SNOW	CINNAMON PEACH-BLUEBERRY COMPOTE
4	**5**	**6**	**7**	**8**	**9**	**10**
PIÑA COLADA CAKE	FROZEN NECTARINE CUSTARD	MOCHA POPCORN	PEACHY RHUBARB RAISIN PIE	CREAMY CAROB PUDDING	TANGY SUMMER COMPOTE	BLACKBERRY PINEAPPLE COBBLER
11	**12**	**13**	**14**	**15**	**16**	**17**
BAKED MAPLE PEACHES	CANTALOUPE POINTS	SNAPPY FRUIT DIP	RASPBERRY NESTS	VANILLA PLUM PIE ★	RASPBERRIES WITH STRAWBERRY SAUCE	SUNSHINE LAYER CAKE
18	**19**	**20**	**21**	**22**	**23**	**24**
PEACHY RHUBARB SAUCE	NO-CRUST BLUEBERRY CHIFFON PIE	PLUM GOOD MERINGUE	PEACH-TOPPED FROZEN ICE MOLD	EXOTIC COMPOTE	CRUNCHY PEACH CRISP	PECAN BARS
25	**26**	**27**	**28**	**29**	**30**	**31**
ALMOND-STUFFED PEACHES	RASPBERRY SORBET	ONE RIPE PLUM	CAROB COCONUT LOAVES	WATERMELON BASKET	CINNAMON CREAM	BLUEBERRY BANANA PIE

168

Crunchy Peach Crisp (page 184)

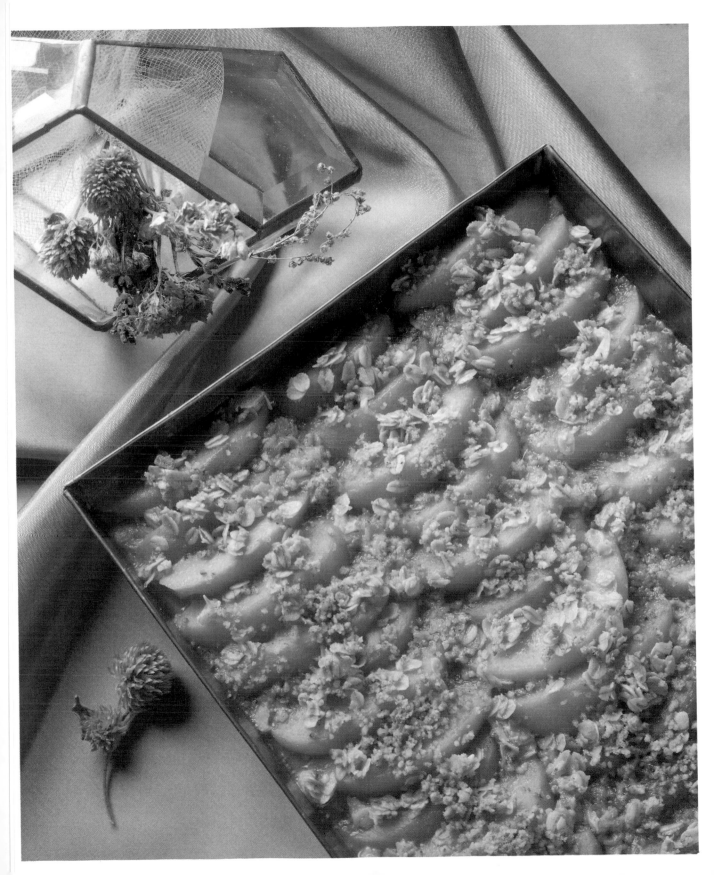

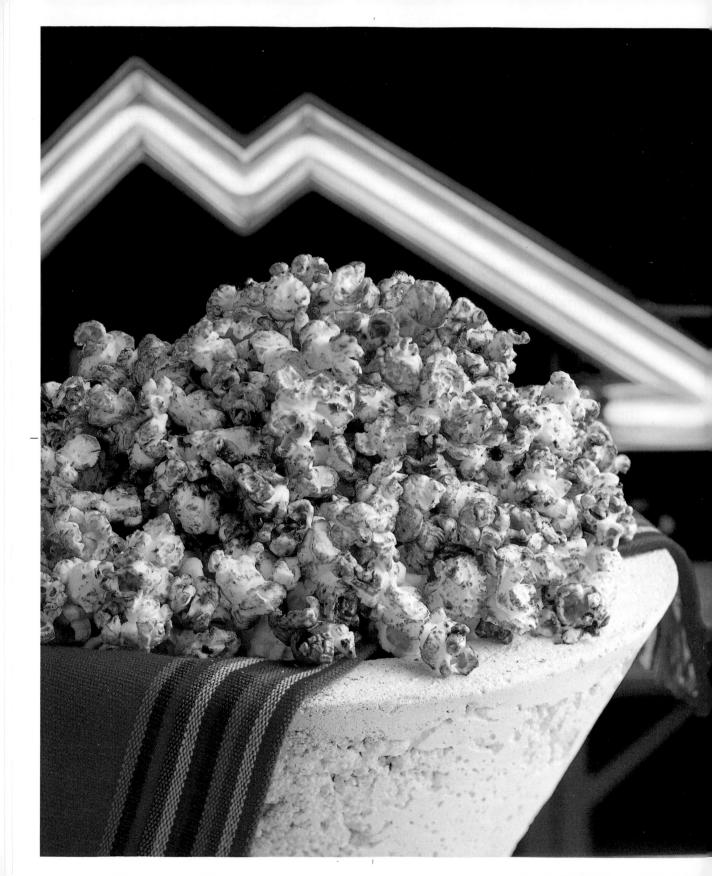

Piña Colada Cake

1 8-ounce can unsweetened
   crushed pineapple
2 teaspoons unflavored gelatin
1 tablespoon honey
1 teaspoon rum extract
½ cup ice water
⅓ cup instant nonfat dry milk
½ cup unsweetened flaked coconut
1 Heavenly Angel Food Cake
   (page 42)

Drain pineapple, reserving juice.

In a small saucepan, sprinkle gelatin over reserved pineapple juice and set aside for 5 minutes to soften. Add honey and cook over medium heat, stirring constantly, until gelatin is completely dissolved. Stir in extract. Chill until thickened but not set.

In a medium-size bowl, beat together ice water and nonfat dry milk until soft peaks form. Beat in gelatin mixture. Fold in pineapple and coconut.

Frost cake with mixture and refrigerate for at least 4 hours before serving.

Makes 8 servings
(144 calories per serving)

Grape Snow

1 envelope unflavored gelatin
1½ cups water, divided
1 tablespoon honey
1 6-ounce can unsweetened
   frozen red or white grape
   juice concentrate
3 egg whites

In a small saucepan, soften gelatin for 5 minutes in ½ cup water. Add honey and heat over low heat, stirring constantly, until gelatin dissolves.

Remove from heat. Stir in remaining water and grape juice concentrate, stirring until grape juice has melted. Chill until mixture is the consistency of unbeaten egg whites, about 1¼ hours.

Transfer grape juice mixture to a large bowl. Add egg whites and beat until mixture is fluffy and thickened. Divide among 8 dessert glasses and refrigerate until set. Keep chilled until ready to serve.

Makes 8 servings
(67 calories per serving)

Mocha Popcorn (page 178)

Sunshine Filling

3 tablespoons cornstarch
2 cups freshly squeezed
   orange juice, divided

2 tablespoons honey
½ teaspoon lemon extract

Shake together cornstarch and ½ cup of the orange juice in a jar with a tight-fitting lid.

Mix together remaining orange juice, honey, and cornstarch mixture in a medium-size saucepan. Bring to a boil over medium heat, stirring constantly, and cook, until thickened. Add lemon extract and allow to cool.

Makes about 2 cups
(15 calories per tablespoon)

Raspberry Nests

1 recipe for Meringue Shells
   (page 84)
2 cups fresh raspberries, divided
½ cup Delicious Diet Cream
   (page 119), divided

Bake Meringue Shells according to directions.

Put ⅓ cup of the raspberries into each Meringue Shell. Top with about a tablespoon of the diet cream and serve immediately.

Makes 6 servings
(42 calories per serving)

Raspberries with Strawberry Sauce

1½ cups Slim Pastry Cream
   (page 270)
1 quart fresh raspberries
¾ cup Strawberry Sauce
   (page 253), divided

Put ¼ cup of the pastry cream into each of 6 dessert dishes. Divide raspberries among the dishes. Top each with 2 tablespoons of the Strawberry Sauce and serve immediately.

Makes 6 servings
(156 calories per serving)

Pecan Bars (page 186)

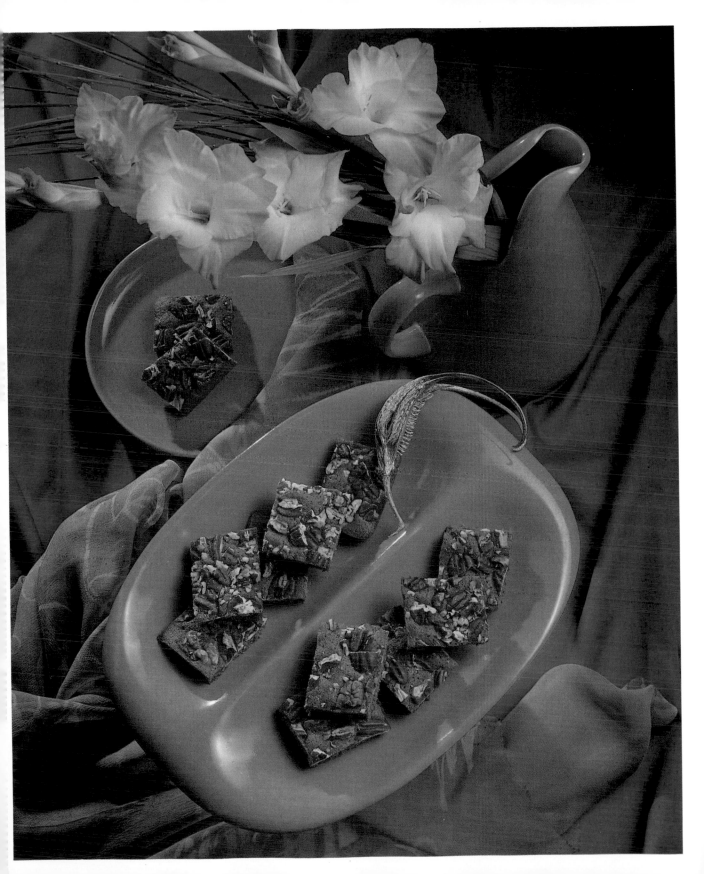

Crunchy Peach Crisp

3½ cups unsweetened frozen
   sliced peaches, thawed and
   drained with juice reserved
2 tablespoons honey, warmed
2 teaspoons freshly squeezed
   lemon juice
¼ teaspoon ground ginger
¾ teaspoon ground cinnamon
½ cup quick-cooking oats
2 tablespoons ground pecans
1 tablespoon butter, softened
1 tablespoon water

Preheat oven to 350°F. Spray an
8 × 8-inch glass baking dish with vegetable spray.

In a medium-size bowl, toss peach
slices with ¼ cup of the reserved juice, 1
tablespoon of the honey, lemon juice,
and spices. Arrange in a layer on bottom
of prepared dish.

In a small bowl, mix together oats,
pecans, remaining honey, butter and
water to soften oats slightly. Spread on
top of peaches. Bake on middle shelf of
oven until peaches are tender, about 25
minutes.

Makes 8 servings
(159 calories per serving)

Exotic Compote

1 fresh pineapple, peeled, cored,
   and cut into chunks
2 seedless oranges, peeled, sectioned, and sections quartered
3 kiwi fruits, peeled and cut into
   wedges
¼ cup freshly squeezed orange
   juice
1 tablespoon freshly squeezed
   lemon juice
1 tablespoon honey, warmed
1 banana

In a large glass bowl, toss together
pineapple, oranges, and kiwis.

In a small bowl, mix together juices
and honey. Toss with fruit in large bowl.

Slice banana. Toss with other ingredients, coating well.

Makes 8 servings
(87 calories per serving)

Snappy Fruit Dip

½ cup plain nonfat yogurt
½ cup sour cream
1 tablespoon honey
1 tablespoon minced crystallized
   ginger
1 tangerine, peeled and sectioned,
   pith removed
¾ cup fresh blackberries
½ cup seedless white grapes

In a small bowl, combine yogurt, sour cream, honey, and ginger. Chill.

When ready to serve, arrange fruit decoratively on a plate around bowl of dip.

Makes 4 servings
(105 calories per serving)

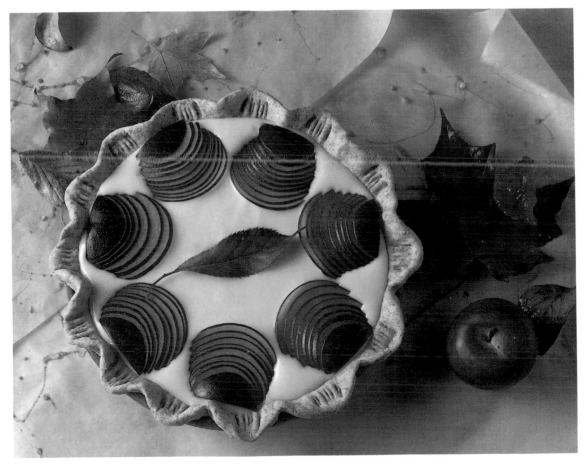

Vanilla Plum Pie (page 179)

Watermelon Basket

This favorite classic is always a crowd pleaser.

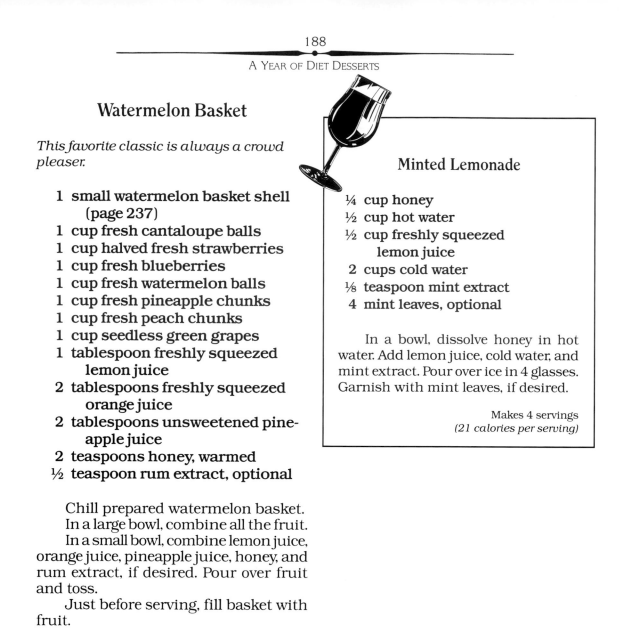

- 1 **small watermelon basket shell (page 237)**
- 1 **cup fresh cantaloupe balls**
- 1 **cup halved fresh strawberries**
- 1 **cup fresh blueberries**
- 1 **cup fresh watermelon balls**
- 1 **cup fresh pineapple chunks**
- 1 **cup fresh peach chunks**
- 1 **cup seedless green grapes**
- 1 **tablespoon freshly squeezed lemon juice**
- 2 **tablespoons freshly squeezed orange juice**
- 2 **tablespoons unsweetened pine-apple juice**
- 2 **teaspoons honey, warmed**
- ½ **teaspoon rum extract, optional**

Chill prepared watermelon basket.
In a large bowl, combine all the fruit.
In a small bowl, combine lemon juice, orange juice, pineapple juice, honey, and rum extract, if desired. Pour over fruit and toss.
Just before serving, fill basket with fruit.

Makes 16 servings
(45 calories per serving)

Minted Lemonade

- ¼ **cup honey**
- ½ **cup hot water**
- ½ **cup freshly squeezed lemon juice**
- 2 **cups cold water**
- ⅛ **teaspoon mint extract**
- 4 **mint leaves, optional**

In a bowl, dissolve honey in hot water. Add lemon juice, cold water, and mint extract. Pour over ice in 4 glasses. Garnish with mint leaves, if desired.

Makes 4 servings
(21 calories per serving)

Cinnamon Cream

2 cups skim milk
1 envelope unflavored gelatin
2 tablespoons honey
1 teaspoon ground cinnamon
2 eggs, separated
6 seedless orange sections
   ground cinnamon for sprinkling

In the top of a double boiler set over simmering water, heat skim milk to scalding. Add gelatin and stir until dissolved. Mix in honey and cinnamon.

In a small bowl, beat egg yolks until thick. Gradually whisk about ¼ cup of the hot milk mixture into egg yolks, then whisk mixture back into remaining hot milk in top of double boiler. Continue cooking until pudding is thick and smooth, stirring constantly. Remove from heat and allow to cool.

In a medium-size bowl, beat egg whites until stiff peaks form. Fold into pudding. Divide among 6 dessert dishes. Top each with an orange section and chill.

Sprinkle with cinnamon just before serving.

Makes 6 servings
(88 calories per serving)

SEPTEMBER

Diet Ideas for
Puddings and Piecrusts

FRUIT OF THE MONTH: **CANTALOUPE**

DESSERT OF THE MONTH: **CANTALOUPE SHERBET**

DRINK OF THE MONTH: **CANTALOUPE COOLER**

				1	Labor Day 2	3
				COLORFUL FRUIT MOLD	LAZY DAY LOAF CAKE	CANTALOUPE SHERBET ★
4	5	6	7	8	9	10
PEACH PEAR SHORTCAKES	PEACH WHIP	SURPRISE FRUIT PUDDING	PLUM EASY TARTS	PRETTY PEACHES	RAISIN SOUFFLÉ	LEMON PUDDING CAKE
11	12	13	14	15	16	17
FRENCH CAROB ICE MILK	APPLESAUCE CUSTARD	ABRACADABRA COCONUT PIE	CAROB CHIP PUDDING	FROZEN FRUITSICLES	BLUEBERRY APPLES	BANANA BITS
18	19	20	21	22	23	24
EASY ORANGE PLUM PUDDING	BLACKBERRY SHORTCAKE	VANILLA POACHED PEACHES	CRUSTLESS LEMON PUMPKIN PIE	BLINCHIKI WITH BLUEBERRY GRAPE SAUCE	BANANA FRAPPE	GINGERBREAD SQUARES
25	26	27	28	29	30	
COCONUT CAROB PUDDING	⅛ RIPE CANTALOUPE	FRESH FIGS WITH CREAMY TOPPING	EVERYDAY SUNDAES	BRANDIED PEACH TAPIOCA	TROPICAL TART	

Blackberry Shortcake (page 206)

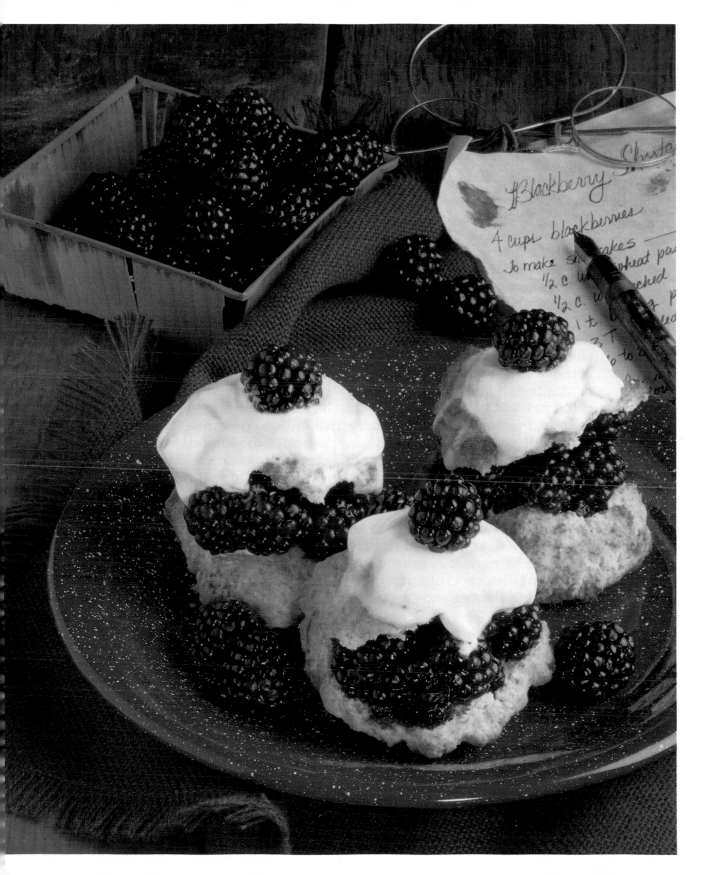

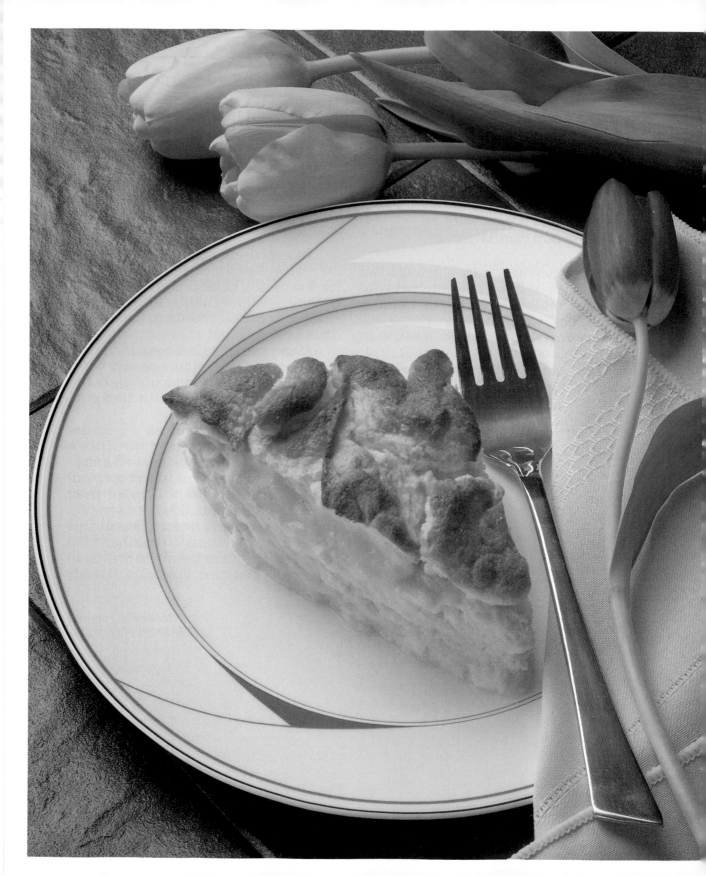

Lemon Pudding Cake

2 eggs, separated
⅛ teaspoon cream of tartar
¾ cup skim milk
3 tablespoons whole wheat pastry
   flour
¼ cup freshly squeezed lemon juice
⅛ teaspoon baking soda
2 tablespoons honey
1 tablespoon butter, melted
1 teaspoon grated lemon peel
½ teaspoon lemon extract

Preheat oven to 350°F. Lightly butter a 1½-quart casserole.

In a medium-size bowl, beat egg whites until foamy. Add cream of tartar and continue beating until stiff peaks form.

In a large bowl, beat egg yolks. Shake together skim milk and flour in a jar with a tight-fitting lid. Beat into egg yolks. Add remaining ingredients and blend well.

Stir a small amount of the yolk mixture into whites to lighten, then fold whites into yolk mixture. Turn into prepared casserole and set in a pan of hot water on bottom shelf of oven. Bake for 55 to 60 minutes.

Makes 4 servings
(138 calories per serving)

Blinchiki with Blueberry Grape Sauce

1 cup skim milk
1 tablespoon freshly squeezed
   lemon juice
1 egg
1 tablespoon butter, melted and
   cooled
1 tablespoon honey
1 teaspoon vanilla extract
1¼ cups whole wheat pastry flour
1 teaspoon baking powder
1½ cups Blueberry Grape Sauce
   (page 134)

In a small bowl, mix together skim milk and lemon juice and set aside for 15 minutes.

In a medium-size bowl, beat together egg, milk mixture, butter, honey, and vanilla.

Sift together flour and baking powder into another small bowl and whisk to blend. Stir into milk mixture just until blended. Chill for 1 hour.

Spray a nonstick skillet with vegetable spray. Heat over medium heat until water dropped into skillet sizzles. Drop batter into skillet, allowing ¼ cup for each blinchiki. Cook until bubbles form, then flip over, and cook on the other side for 30 seconds.

Serve topped with Blueberry Grape Sauce.

Makes 6 servings
(178 calories per serving)

Lemon Pudding Cake (on this page)

Vanilla Poached Peaches

Since the poaching water is discarded, you get the sweetness of the honey while avoiding most of the calories.

    2 cups water
    ½ cup honey
    ½ vanilla bean, split lengthwise
    4 large fresh peaches, halved,
         peeled, and pitted
    1 cup Ruby Raspberry Sauce
         (page 139), divided
   24 fresh raspberries

In a large saucepan, combine water, honey, and vanilla bean. Bring to a boil, stirring occasionally. Reduce heat, add peaches, cover, and cook 4 minutes. (Water should be barely simmering.) With a slotted spoon, turn peach halves over. Continue to poach until peaches are tender but not mushy, about 4 more minutes.

Carefully remove peaches to a plate. Discard poaching water. Cover peaches with plastic wrap and chill.

At serving time, spoon 1 tablespoon of the Ruby Raspberry Sauce onto each of 8 individual dessert plates. Top sauce with a peach half, spoon another tablespoon of sauce over peach, and decorate with 3 raspberries.

Makes 8 servings
(104 calories per serving)

Gingerbread Squares

    2 tablespoons butter, softened
    2 tablespoons honey
    1 tablespoon molasses
    2 eggs
    ¼ cup skim milk
    1 cup whole wheat pastry flour
    ½ teaspoon baking powder
    1 teaspoon ground ginger
    1 teaspoon ground cinnamon
    ¼ teaspoon ground nutmeg
    ¼ cup raisins, plumped

Preheat oven to 350°F. Spray an 8 × 8-inch pan with vegetable spray.

In a large bowl, cream together butter, honey, and molasses. Beat in eggs and skim milk.

In a medium-size bowl, whisk together flour, baking powder, ginger, cinnamon, and nutmeg. Drain raisins and toss them with 1 tablespoon of flour mixture. Mix remaining flour mixture into moist ingredients. Fold in raisins. Spread batter in prepared pan and bake on middle shelf of oven for 15 minutes.

Cut into 9 squares. Cool on wire rack.

Makes 9 servings
(119 calories per serving)

Vanilla Poached Peaches (on this page)

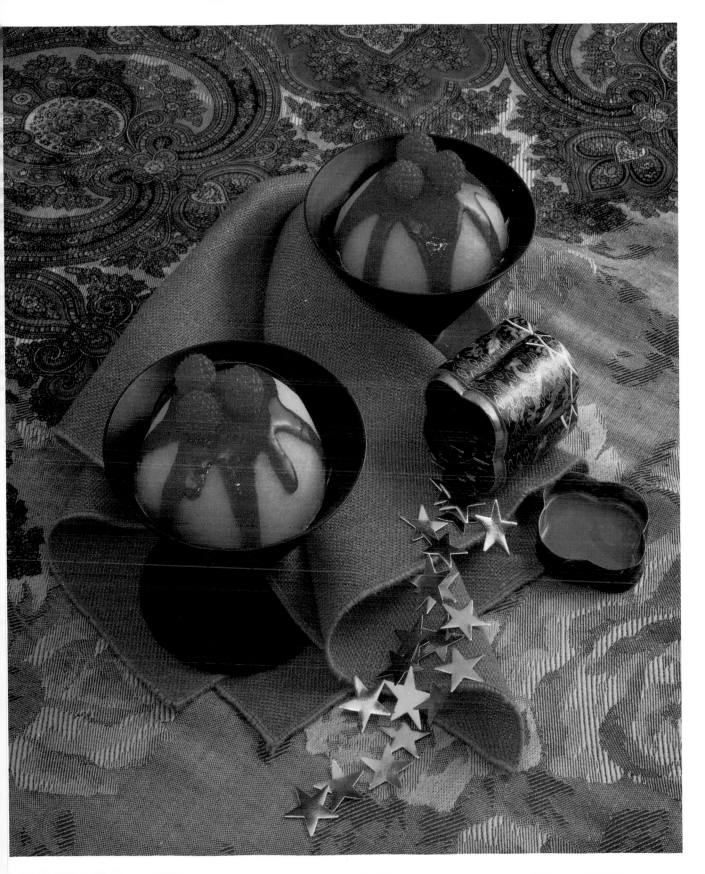

Crustless Lemon Pumpkin Pie

3 eggs
1¼ cups pumpkin puree
¾ cup skim milk
⅓ cup plus 2 tablespoons honey
1 teaspoon ground cinnamon
¼ teaspoon ground ginger
¼ teaspoon ground nutmeg
1 cup plain nonfat yogurt
2 teaspoons grated lemon rind

Preheat oven to 350°F. Spray a 9-inch pie plate with vegetable spray.

In a large bowl, beat together eggs, pumpkin, skim milk, ⅓ cup of the honey, cinnamon, ginger, and nutmeg. Turn into prepared pie plate and bake on middle shelf of oven until a knife inserted near the center comes out clean, 50 to 55 minutes. Allow to cool.

In a small bowl, gently combine yogurt and remaining honey. Spread on top of pie. Chill.

Sprinkle with grated lemon rind, and serve immediately.

Makes 8 servings
(84 calories per serving)

Fresh Figs with Creamy Topping

Figs should be used on the day they're purchased. They are oh, so perishable!

8 fresh figs
¾ cup evaporated skim milk, chilled
2 tablespoons honey
1 teaspoon vanilla extract
¼ teaspoon ground cinnamon
4 mint leaves, optional

Put 2 figs into each of 4 dessert dishes.

In a medium-size bowl, beat evaporated milk until foamy. Add honey, vanilla, and cinnamon and beat until the consistency of whipped cream. Divide among dessert dishes, mounding on top of figs. Decorate with mint leaves, if desired.

Makes 4 servings
(150 calories per serving)

Blackberry Shortcake

6 Skinny Shortcakes (page 79)
4 cups fresh blackberries
¾ cup Delicious Diet Cream (page 119), divided

Cut shortcakes into halves crosswise. Divide berries among shortcakes, mounding them on bottom halves. Put tops over berries. Top each with 2 tablespoons of the diet cream.

Makes 6 servings
(193 calories per serving)

Surprise Fruit Pudding

1 20-ounce can unsweetened
  crushed pineapple
3 envelopes unflavored gelatin
2 tablespoons honey
1½ cups fresh strawberries,
  quartered
½ cup unsweetened flaked
  coconut
½ cup carob chips

Drain pineapple well, reserving juice. In a medium-size saucepan, sprinkle gelatin over reserved juice. Set aside for 5 minutes to soften. Stir in honey and heat over low heat, stirring constantly, until gelatin is dissolved.

Stir in pineapple, strawberries, and coconut. Divide among 8 dessert dishes and sprinkle each with 1 tablespoon carob chips. Chill thoroughly.

Makes 8 servings
(153 calories per serving)

Brandied Peach Tapioca

3 tablespoons quick-cooking
  tapioca
2 cups skim milk
2 tablespoons maple syrup
½ teaspoon ground cinnamon
1 egg yolk, beaten
½ teaspoon brandy extract
½ teaspoon vanilla extract
3 cups unsweetened frozen
  peaches, thawed and drained

In a medium-size saucepan, sprinkle tapioca over skim milk. Set aside for 5 minutes.

Stir in maple syrup, cinnamon, and egg yolk. Bring to a boil over medium heat, stirring constantly. Remove from heat and stir in extracts. When slightly cooled, fold in peaches. Refrigerate until ready to serve.

Makes 8 servings
(98 calories per serving)

Banana Frappe

2 ripe bananas, chunked
1 tablespoon honey
2 cups skim milk
1 teaspoon vanilla extract
½ teaspoon ground cinnamon

In a food processor, puree bananas. Add remaining ingredients and process until blended. Pour into glasses and serve immediately.

Makes 4 servings
(110 calories per serving)

Peach Whip

1 envelope unflavored gelatin
½ cup water
2 tablespoons honey
1 cup peach puree (2 to 3 medium-
　size fresh peaches, peeled and
　pureed in a food processor)
1 teaspoon freshly squeezed
　lemon juice
2 egg whites, at room temperature
⅛ teaspoon cream of tartar

In a small saucepan, sprinkle gelatin over water. Set aside for 5 minutes to soften. Heat over medium heat, stirring constantly, until gelatin dissolves. Remove from heat. Stir in honey, peach puree, and lemon juice. Chill until thickened but not set, stirring occasionally, about 30 minutes.

In a medium-size bowl, beat egg whites until foamy. Add cream of tartar and continue beating until stiff peaks form. Fold into gelatin mixture and chill until set.

Makes 6 servings
(60 calories per serving)

Abracadabra Coconut Pie

It's magic! This tasty treat forms a crust as it bakes.

2 cups skim milk
4 eggs
¼ cup honey
2 tablespoons maple syrup
½ cup whole wheat pastry flour
3 tablespoons butter, cut into pieces
1 teaspoon vanilla extract
¾ cup unsweetened flaked coconut

Preheat oven to 350°F. Spray a 9-inch pie plate with vegetable spray.

In a blender, combine skim milk, eggs, honey, maple syrup, flour, butter, and vanilla. Process until smooth. Stir in coconut. Turn into prepared pie plate and bake on middle shelf of oven until a knife inserted near center comes out clean, about 50 minutes. Serve chilled.

Makes 10 servings
(155 calories per serving)

Easy Orange Plum Pudding

3 tablespoons cornstarch
2 cups freshly squeezed orange
    juice
3 tablespoons honey
4 fresh plums

In a medium-size saucepan, dissolve cornstarch in orange juice. Mix in honey and cook over medium heat, stirring constantly, until thickened, about 15 minutes.

Pit plums and cut into eighths. Stir into orange juice mixture. Turn into a medium-size bowl and chill.

Makes 6 servings
(111 calories per serving)

OCTOBER

The Proper Care, Storage, and Freezing of Desserts

				1	2	3
FRUIT OF THE MONTH: **PINEAPPLE** *DESSERT OF THE MONTH:* **TROPICAL PINEAPPLE DELIGHT** *DRINK OF THE MONTH:* **ORANGE PINEAPPLE PUNCH**				FAUX CAFE WHIP	ONE SLICE FRESH PINEAPPLE	SPICY PUMPKIN CUSTARD
4	**5**	**6**	*Rosh Hashanah* 7	**8**	**9**	**10**
PEPPERMINT ALASKA	PRETTY STRAWBERRY BAVARIAN	LEMON CHIFFON PIE	ROSH HASHANAH CARROT CAKE	VANILLA CREAM WITH RASPBERRY SAUCE	APPLE RAISIN TART	FRESH PINEAPPLE SORBET
11	*Columbus Day* 12	**13**	**14**	**15**	*Yom Kippur* 16	**17**
RAISIN RICE CHEWS	DISCOVERY CAKE	LEMELON	CRAN-PINEAPPLE PIE	SNOW PUDDING WITH CUSTARD SAUCE	YOM KIPPUR DATE NUT CAKE	TROPICAL PINEAPPLE DELIGHT ★
18	**19**	**20**	**21**	**22**	**23**	**24**
STUFFED DATES	CRANBERRY PINEAPPLE FLUFF	CAMOCHA PIE	GRAPEFRUIT GRANITA	BAKED PRUNE WHIP	LIME-GLAZED BAKED PINEAPPLE	UPPER CRUST LEMON CUSTARD PIE
25	**26**	**27**	**28**	**29**	**30**	*Halloween* 31
ORANGE CAROB WHIP	OCTOBER CAKE	AUTUMN SUNDAE	ORANGE WHIP	COOL PINEAPPLE CREPES	COMPANY APPLES	PUMPKIN CUPCAKES

210

Pumpkin Cupcakes (page 230)

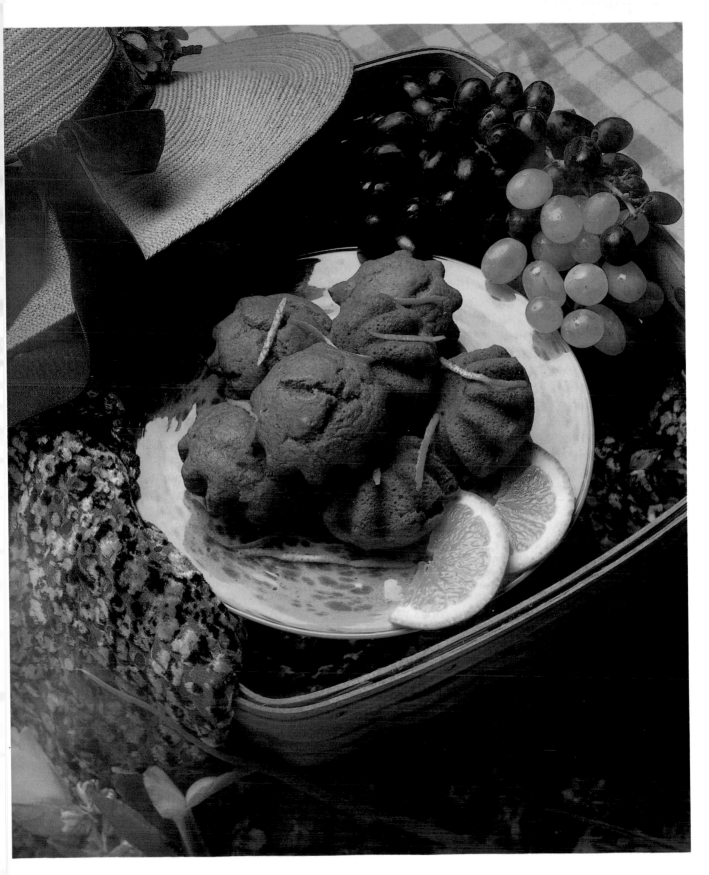

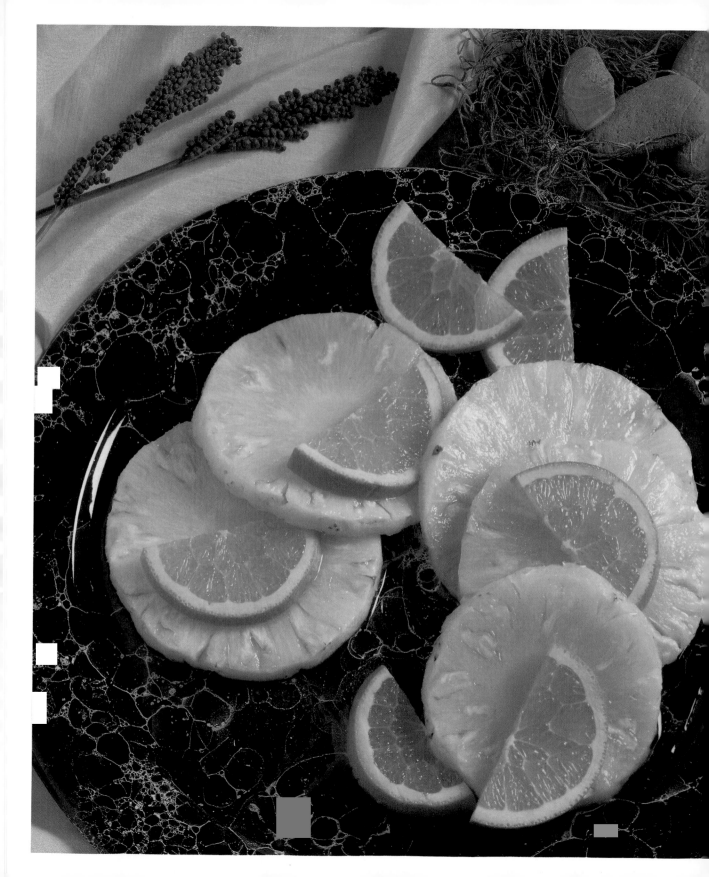

Apple Raisin Tart

1 recipe for Mini Piecrust
   (page 113)
4 medium-size apples
1 tablespoon freshly squeezed
   lemon juice
2 tablespoons cornstarch
1 4½-ounce jar strained peaches
¼ cup raisins
¼ cup honey
1½ teaspoons ground cinnamon

Preheat oven to 400°F. Line a 9-inch pie plate with piecrust according to directions and set aside.

Peel, core, and thinly slice apples into a large bowl. Mix in lemon juice.

In a small bowl, dissolve cornstarch in strained peaches. Add to apple mixture. Add raisins, honey, and cinnamon, tossing to blend well. Turn into pie shell and bake on bottom shelf of oven for 15 minutes. Turn oven down to 375°F and bake until apples are soft and lightly browned, about 30 minutes more.

Makes 10 servings
(120 calories per serving)

Faux Cafe Whip

A summertime treat for coffee lovers.

1 envelope unflavored gelatin
2½ teaspoons decaffeinated instant
   coffee
⅓ cup honey
1¾ cups boiling water
1½ teaspoons vanilla extract

In a medium-size bowl, dissolve gelatin, coffee, and honey together in boiling water. Add vanilla extract and chill until thick but not set.

Beat until volume doubles. Divide among 4 dessert dishes and chill until set.

Makes 4 servings
(91 calories per serving)

Stuffed Dates

12 pitted dates
¼ cup Reduced Calorie Peanut
   Butter (page 59), divided
¼ cup Coconut Sugar (page 66)

Stuff each date with 1 teaspoon of the peanut butter. Roll in Coconut Sugar.

Makes 4 servings
(156 calories per serving)

Lime-Glazed Baked Pineapple (page 228)

Yom Kippur Date Nut Cake

3 eggs
⅓ cup honey
1 teaspoon vanilla extract
⅓ cup whole wheat pastry flour
⅓ cup unbleached white flour
1 teaspoon baking powder
½ cup chopped dates
¼ cup chopped pecans

Preheat oven to 350°F. Spray an 8 × 8-inch pan with vegetable spray.

In a large bowl, beat together eggs and honey for 5 minutes. Beat in vanilla.

Sift together whole wheat pastry flour, unbleached white flour, and baking powder into a small bowl. In another small bowl, toss dates and nuts with 2 tablespoons of the flour mixture. Fold the rest of the flour into egg mixture. Fold in dates and nuts.

Turn into prepared pan and bake on middle shelf of oven for 25 minutes.

Cool in pan. Cut into 9 squares.

Makes 9 servings
(148 calories per serving)

Camocha Pie

To make this dessert even lower in calories, spray pie plate with vegetable spray and eliminate the crust.

1 recipe for Carob Cookie Crust (page 225)
2 eggs
1½ cups low-fat cottage cheese
¾ cup evaporated skim milk
2 teaspoons cornstarch
½ cup honey
1 teaspoon decaffeinated instant coffee
1 tablespoon vanilla extract

Preheat oven to 350°F.

Prepare piecrust according to directions.

In a food processor, blend remaining ingredients until smooth. Pour over piecrust and bake on middle shelf of oven until firm, about 40 minutes.

Makes 12 servings
(86 calories per serving)

Autumn Sundae (page 230)

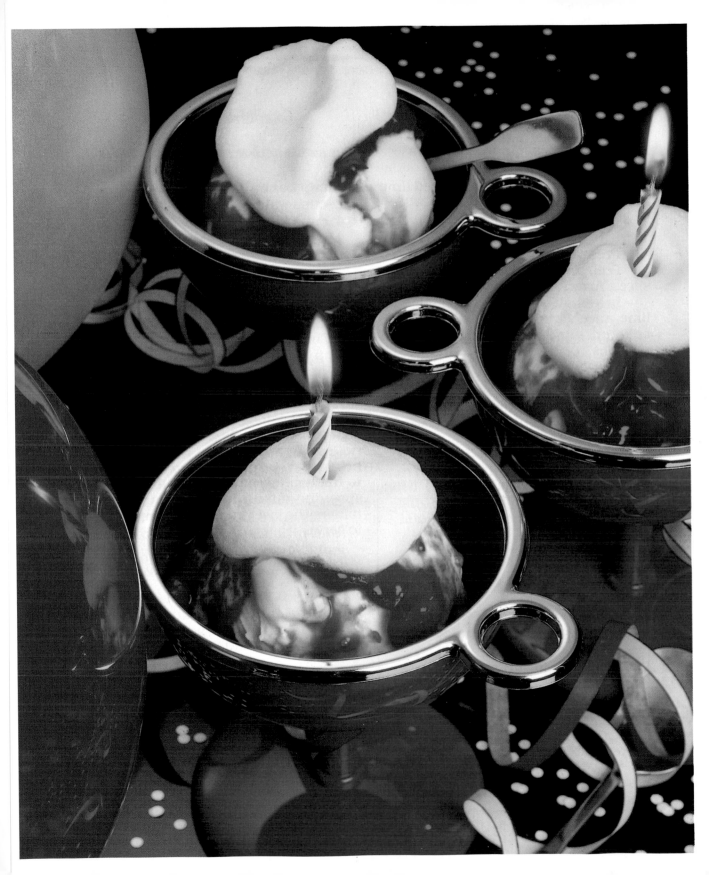

October Cake

1 recipe for Jelly Roll Cake
   (page 54)
1 cup low-fat cottage cheese
¼ cup maple syrup
⅓ cup pureed cooked pumpkin
2 teaspoons vanilla extract
½ teaspoon ground cinnamon

Bake cake according to directions.
In a food processor, blend remaining
ingredients. Refrigerate until thickened.
Cut cake in half, crosswise. Spread
half of pumpkin frosting on 1 half. Top
with second half of cake and spread with
remaining frosting. Refrigerate until
ready to serve.

Makes 12 servings
(171 calories per serving)

Autumn Sundae

2 cups Vanilla Ice Milk (page 79),
   divided
1 cup Cranberry Applesauce
   (page 268), divided
¼ cup Mock Whipped Cream
   (page 10), divided, optional

Divide ice milk among 4, long-
stemmed dessert glasses. Top each with
¼ cup of the Cranberry Applesauce and
1 tablespoon of the Mock Whipped
Cream, if desired. Serve immediately.

Makes 4 servings
(149 calories per serving)

Pumpkin Cupcakes

½ cup whole wheat pastry flour
½ cup unbleached white flour
½ teaspoon baking soda
½ teaspoon baking powder
1½ teaspoons ground cinnamon
½ teaspoon ground allspice
2 eggs
⅓ cup honey
2 teaspoons molasses
2 tablespoons vegetable oil
¼ cup skim milk
½ cup pureed cooked pumpkin
1 teaspoon vanilla extract
72 raisins, optional
12 small Orange Fans (page 235),
   optional

Preheat oven to 350°F. Spray a
12-cup muffin tin with vegetable spray.
Sift together whole wheat pastry
flour, unbleached white flour, baking
soda, baking powder, cinnamon, and
allspice into a medium-size bowl.
In a large bowl, beat eggs until light
colored. Beat in remaining ingredients.
Mix in dry ingredients and divide among
prepared muffin cups. Bake on middle
shelf of oven for 15 to 20 minutes.
Decorate, if desired, and cool on
wire racks.

Makes 12 servings
(116 calories per serving)

Company Apples

5 McIntosh apples
  ground cinnamon for sprinkling
4 egg whites
¼ teaspoon cream of tartar
1 teaspoon vanilla extract

Preheat oven to 350°F. Spray a large shallow baking dish with vegetable spray.

Core, but do not peel, apples, cutting them into halves from top to bottom. Place, cut side up, in prepared dish. Sprinkle with cinnamon and bake on middle shelf of oven until fork tender, 25 to 30 minutes.

In a medium-size bowl, beat egg whites until foamy. Add cream of tartar and continue beating until stiff peaks form. Beat in vanilla.

Spoon meringue on tops of baked apples. Increase heat to 400°F and return apples to oven until meringue is golden brown, about 5 minutes. Serve warm.

Makes 10 servings
(55 calories per serving)

Orange Whip

2 eggs, separated
2 cups skim milk
½ envelope unflavored gelatin
¼ cup honey
2 teaspoons orange extract
6 mint leaves, optional

In a small bowl, beat egg yolks until fluffy.

In the top of a double boiler, mix together egg yolks and skim milk. Sprinkle gelatin over top and set aside for 5 minutes to soften. Stir in honey and cook over low heat, stirring constantly, until gelatin has dissolved and mixture has thickened slightly. Remove from heat and stir in orange extract. Chill until thickened but not set.

In a medium-size bowl, beat egg whites until stiff. Fold into orange gelatin. Divide among 6 long-stemmed dessert glasses and chill until set.

Just before serving, decorate with mint leaves, if desired.

Makes 6 servings
(102 calories per serving)

NOVEMBER

Decorating Desserts with Diet in Mind

				1	2	3
FRUIT OF THE MONTH: **PRUNES** DESSERT OF THE MONTH: **PRUNE BARS** DRINK OF THE MONTH: **CRANBERRY DELIGHT**				FROZEN PUMPKIN DESSERT	CHINESE MANDARIN ALMOND CUSTARD	AUTUMN FRUIT MEDLEY
4 PRUNE BARS ★	**5** MANDARIN KABOBS	**6** PERSIMMON PUDDING	**7** TOPLESS APPLE CRANBERRY PIE	**8** LEMON CAKE ROLL	**9** CAROB COFFEE TREAT SUPREME	**10** SAUCY CREPES
11 PEPPERMINT MERINGUE PIE	**12** TWO-GRAPEFRUIT TREAT	**13** HONEY CHEESE PIE	**14** CRANBERRY NUT CAKES	**15** COCONUT SOUFFLÉ	**16** FRENCH PEPPERMINT ICE MILK	**17** BANANA TAPIOCA
18 SURPRISE PEANUTTY VANILLA PIE	**19** FRESH ORANGE GELATIN	**20** THREE COOKED PRUNES	**21** MOLASSES GINGER JOYS	**22** INDIVIDUAL BRANDY SOUFFLÉS WITH STRAWBERRY SAUCE	**23** ORANGE BANANA POPS	**24** APPLE PEAR SCALLOP
25 INDIAN PUDDING	*Thanksgiving* **26** PUMPKIN PINEAPPLE PIE	**27** HAYSTACKS	**28** CREAMY / CAROB CHIP CHEESECAKE	**29** FLUFFY GRAPE DESSERT	**30** GREEK YOGURT PRUNE PIE	

Cranberry Nut Cakes (page 247)

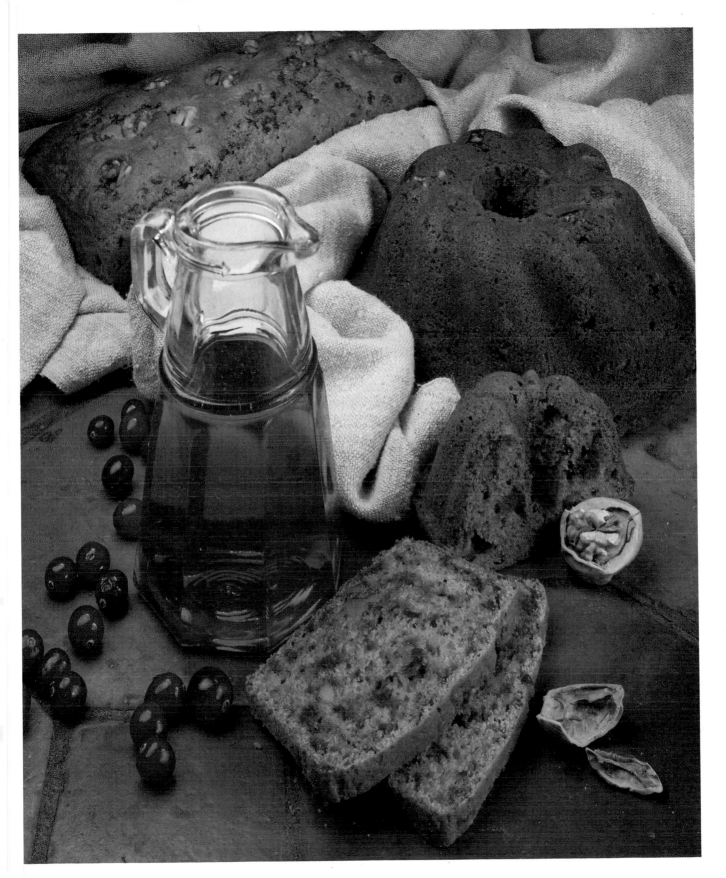

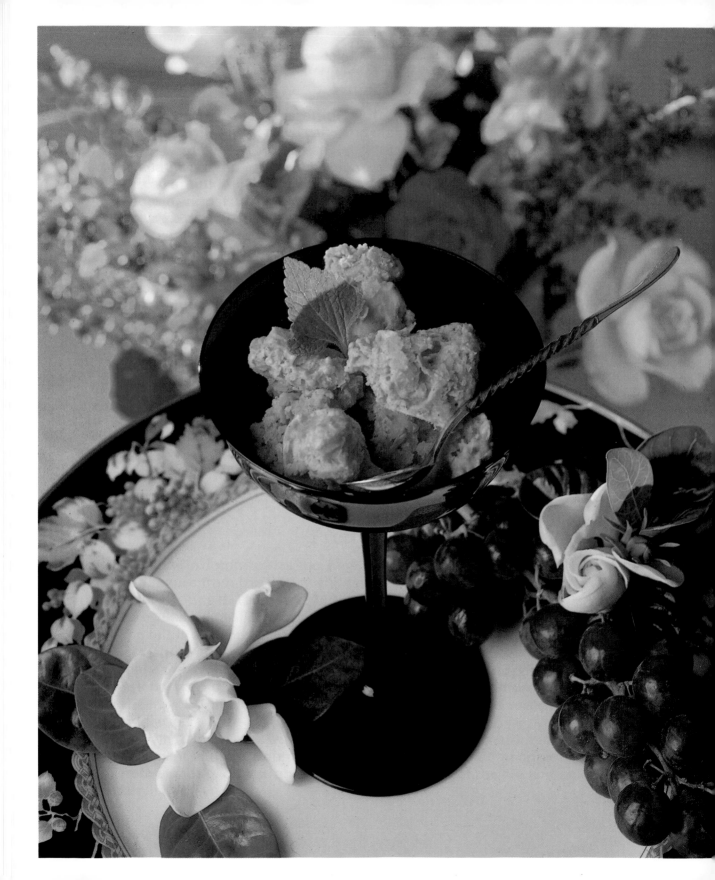

Autumn Fruit Medley

1 tablespoon honey
1 teaspoon freshly squeezed
   lemon juice
1 tablespoon water
1 seedless orange
1 large apple
1 ripe banana
1 Bosc pear
16 seedless green or red grapes,
   halved

In a small bowl, mix together honey, lemon juice, and water.

Peel and section orange. Quarter sections and place them into a glass bowl. Core, but do not peel, apple. Cut it into chunks and add to bowl, tossing with orange pieces. Cut banana into rounds. Halve rounds and add to other fruit, tossing. Peel and core pear. Cut into chunks and toss with other fruit. Add grapes and honey mixture, tossing to coat well. Chill until serving time.

Makes 8 servings
(60 calories per serving)

★ Prune Bars

1 cup pitted prunes
1 cup plus 1 tablespoon whole
   wheat pastry flour, divided
¾ cup apple juice
2 tablespoons butter
1 tablespoon honey
1 teaspoon baking powder
½ teaspoon baking soda
1 teaspoon ground cinnamon
¼ teaspoon ground nutmeg
1 egg
2 tablespoons chopped pecans,
   optional

Preheat oven to 350°F. Spray an 8 × 8-inch pan with vegetable spray.

In a food processor, chop prunes with 1 tablespoon of the flour. Put into a small saucepan with apple juice and butter. Bring to a boil, stirring constantly, until butter melts. Mix in honey. Pour into a large bowl and allow to cool slightly.

Sift flour, baking powder, baking soda, cinnamon, and nutmeg into a medium-size bowl. Whisk to blend. Stir into prune mixture.

Beat egg and stir into batter. Fold in nuts, if desired, and turn into prepared pan. Bake on middle shelf of oven for 25 to 30 minutes.

Allow to cool in pan. Cut into 16 pieces.

Makes 16 bars
(80 calories per bar)

Frozen Pumpkin Dessert (page 241)

Tangy Lemon Filling

3 tablespoons cornstarch
⅓ cup freshly squeezed
    lemon juice
1 cup water

¼ cup honey
1 egg yolk
1 teaspoon butter

In a jar with a tight-fitting lid, shake together cornstarch and lemon juice, or whisk in a small bowl until thoroughly blended. Pour into a small saucepan. Add water and honey and cook over medium heat, stirring constantly, until mixture thickens.

In a small bowl, whisk egg yolk. Pour some of the hot lemon mixture into egg yolk, whisking constantly. Return to saucepan and continue cooking, stirring constantly, for 2 minutes. Remove from heat and stir in butter. Cool before using. (Filling will thicken as it cools.)

Makes about 1½ cups
(19 calories per tablespoon)

Carob Coffee Treat Supreme

¾ cup decaffeinated coffee, cooled
¼ cup water
3 tablespoons honey
1 envelope unflavored gelatin
8 Carob Thins (page 55)
3 egg whites
¼ teaspoon cream of tartar
1½ teaspoons vanilla extract

In a small saucepan, combine coffee, water, and honey. Sprinkle gelatin over mixture and set aside to soften for 5 minutes. Heat, stirring constantly, over medium heat until gelatin dissolves. Pour into a medium-size bowl and chill, stirring occasionally, until mixture is thick but not set.

Break cookies into small pieces and fold into gelatin.

In another medium-size bowl, beat egg whites until foamy. Sprinkle in cream of tartar and vanilla and continue beating until stiff peaks form. Fold into gelatin and chill until set.

Makes 6 servings
(85 calories per serving)

Saucy Crepes

1 cup Applesauce (page 90)
½ teaspoon ground cinnamon
8 warm Delicious Diet Crepes
    (page 33)
½ cup plain low-fat yogurt
1 tablespoon honey
½ teaspoon vanilla extract
    ground cinnamon for sprinkling

In a small saucepan, heat together applesauce and cinnamon. Spread 2 tablespoons of the mixture on each crepe and roll up.

In a small bowl, gently whisk together yogurt, honey, and vanilla. Top each crepe with 1 tablespoon of the mixture. Sprinkle with cinnamon and serve immediately.

Makes 8 servings
(71 calories per serving)

Persimmon Pudding

This delicate pudding has a custard base.

3 eggs
1 cup evaporated skim milk
½ teaspoon ground cinnamon
2 cups unsweetened persimmon
    pulp*

In a large bowl, beat eggs slightly.

Heat evaporated skim milk in a small saucepan to scalding. Stir in cinnamon. Slowly whisk into beaten eggs. Stir in persimmon pulp and divide among 9 ovenproof 8-ounce dessert dishes. Set dishes in a large shallow pan and put pan on middle shelf of oven. Pour enough hot water into pan to almost reach the tops of the dishes. Bake for about 40 minutes, or until knife inserted near centers comes out clean.

Makes 9 servings
(75 calories per serving)

*Found in specialty foods stores.

Peppermint Meringue Pie

1 recipe for Meringue Pie Shell
    (page 117)
4 cups French Peppermint Ice Milk
    (page 250)
1 cup seedless red grapes

Bake pie shell according to directions. Allow to cool.

At serving time, fill cooled meringue shell with scoops of ice milk. Decorate with grapes and slice. Serve at once.

Makes 10 servings
(86 calories per serving)

Banana Tapioca

1 recipe for Fluffy Almond Tapioca
    (page 89)
1 ripe banana, coarsely chopped
¼ cup raisins, plumped
¼ teaspoon ground cinnamon

In a medium-size bowl, gently combine all ingredients and serve.

Makes 6 servings
(135 calories per serving)

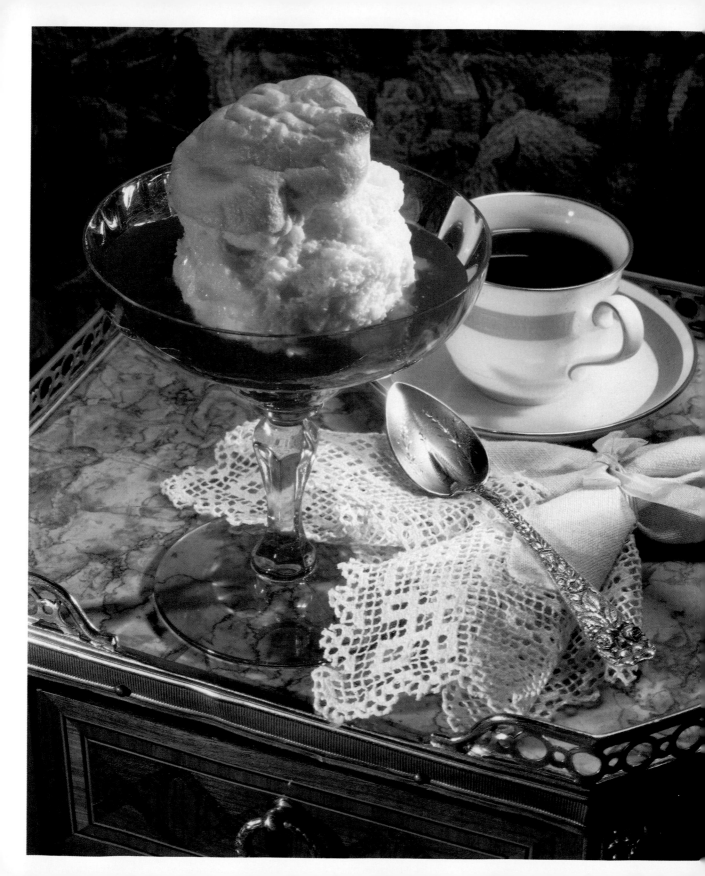

Cranberry Nut Cakes

These loaves freeze nicely and are handy to have for those times when unexpected visitors arrive.

1¼ cups whole wheat pastry flour
1 cup unbleached white flour
1 teaspoon baking powder
1 teaspoon baking soda
⅔ cup honey
⅓ cup vegetable oil
1 cup buttermilk
2 eggs
1 teaspoon orange extract
1½ cups chopped fresh cranberries
¼ cup chopped walnuts

Preheat oven to 350°F. Lightly butter and flour 2 9 × 5-inch loaf pans.

In a large bowl, sift together whole wheat pastry flour, unbleached white flour, baking powder, and baking soda. Add honey, oil, buttermilk, eggs, and orange extract and mix well with a wooden spoon. Mix in cranberries and nuts.

Divide between prepared pans and bake on middle shelf of oven for 40 to 45 minutes, or until a cake tester inserted in centers comes out clean.

Allow to cool in pans for 10 minutes, then turn out onto wire racks to cool completely. Slice each loaf into 10 slices, then halve each slice.

Makes 20 servings per loaf
(138 calories per serving)

Topless Apple Cranberry Pie

1 recipe for Skinny Piecrust (page 6)
6 apples
8 cups water
1 tablespoon freshly squeezed lemon juice
1½ cups fresh cranberries
3 tablespoons honey
1 tablespoon cornstarch
2 teaspoons ground cinnamon

Preheat oven to 400°F. Line bottom and sides of a 10-inch pie plate with pastry, crimping edges, and bake according to directions.

Peel, core, and thinly slice apples, dropping them into water mixed with lemon juice to prevent discoloration.

Drain apples and toss with remaining ingredients. Turn into prepared piecrust. Loosely cover pie with foil and bake on lowest shelf of oven for 30 minutes. Pull foil away from edge of piecrust (keep filling covered) and continue to bake until apples are fork tender, about 20 more minutes. Serve warm or cold.

Makes 10 servings
(127 calories per serving)

Individual Brandy Soufflés with Strawberry Sauce (page 252)

Lemon Cake Roll

This slightly tart dessert is a wonderfully satisfying finale to a light dinner.

> 5 eggs
> ⅓ cup honey
> 1 tablespoon freshly squeezed lemon juice
> 2 teaspoons vanilla extract
> ½ cup whole wheat pastry flour
> ½ cup unbleached white flour
> 1½ cups Tangy Lemon Filling (page 244)

Preheat oven to 275°F. Line bottom of a 15½ × 10½-inch jelly roll pan with parchment paper.

In a large bowl, beat eggs. Add honey, lemon juice, and vanilla and continue beating until eggs thicken, about 10 minutes.

Into a medium-size bowl, sift together whole wheat pastry flour, and unbleached white flour, whisking to blend. Remeasure 1 cup and gradually sift into egg mixture, beating constantly. Pour batter into prepared pan, spreading evenly to sides and smoothing top with spatula. Bake on middle shelf of oven until top springs back when lightly pressed with finger, about 20 minutes.

While cake is baking, spread a tea towel on a flat surface. Put waxed paper on top of it. Turn baked cake out onto lined towel. Remove parchment paper. Trim off edges of cake and roll cake up in lined towel until cool.

Unroll cake, remove towel and waxed paper, spread with Tangy Lemon Filling, and then roll cake up without towel.

Makes 10 servings
(166 calories per serving)

Two-Grapefruit Treat

> 1 seedless pink grapefruit
> 1 seedless white grapefruit
> ½ cup freshly squeezed orange juice
> ½ cup white grape juice
> ¼ cup unsweetened flaked coconut, divided

Peel and section grapefruits. Cut sections into halves, reserving juice in a medium-size bowl. Mix orange juice, grape juice, and reserved grapefruit juice together. Toss with grapefruit sections and chill to mingle flavors.

To serve, divide among 4 dessert dishes and sprinkle each with 1 tablespoon of the coconut.

Makes 4 servings
(98 calories per serving)

Fresh Orange Gelatin

> 1 cup freshly squeezed orange juice
> 1 cup water, divided
> 1 envelope unflavored gelatin
> 1 tablespoon honey
> ¼ teaspoon orange extract

In a medium-size bowl, combine orange juice and ½ cup water.

In a small saucepan, sprinkle gelatin over remaining water. Set aside for 5 minutes to soften. Add honey and heat over medium heat stirring constantly, until gelatin dissolves. Add to juice. Mix in orange extract and chill until set.

Makes 4 servings
(50 calories per serving)

Surprise Peanutty Vanilla Pie

The surprise is the luscious layer of Reduced Calorie peanut butter on the bottom of this dessert.

1 recipe for Skinny Piecrust
   (page 6)
2 tablespoons Reduced Calorie
   Peanut Butter (page 59),
   thinned with water if necessary
2 cups Very Vanilla Pudding
   (page 84)

Line a 9-inch pie plate with pastry and bake according to directions. Set aside to cool.

Spread peanut butter on bottom of cooled crust. Fill with vanilla pudding which has cooled but isn't set. Chill until serving time.

Makes 8 servings
(135 calories per serving)

Orange Banana Pops

1 cup freshly squeezed orange
   juice
1 medium-size ripe banana, cut
   into chunks
1 tablespoon freshly squeezed
   lemon juice

In a food processor, puree together all ingredients. Measure puree and add enough water to make 2 cups, mixing in well. Pour into 8 2-ounce pop molds and freeze.

Makes 8 pops
(28 calories per pop)

Coconut Soufflé

2 eggs
½ cup evaporated skim milk
¼ cup maple syrup
1½ cups low-fat cottage cheese
2 teaspoons vanilla extract
½ cup unsweetened flaked
   coconut
4 egg whites
¼ teaspoon cream of tartar
1 tablespoon honey

Preheat oven to 350°F. Spray a 1½-quart casserole with vegetable spray.

In a blender, blend together eggs, evaporated skim milk, and maple syrup. Add cottage cheese, vanilla, and coconut and blend for about 1 minute.

In a large bowl, beat egg whites until foamy. Add cream of tartar and, while beating, drizzle in honey. Continue beating until stiff peaks form. Fold in cheese mixture and turn into prepared casserole. Set casserole in a large shallow pan and place on middle shelf of oven. Fill pan with enough hot water to reach a depth of 1 inch. Bake for about 30 minutes, or until top of casserole is golden and puffy. Place foil lightly over top and continue baking another 20 minutes. Serve immediately.

Makes 10 servings
(102 calories per serving)

French Peppermint Ice Milk

The addition of an egg is what makes this a French-type ice milk.

  1 **egg**
  ¼ **cup honey**
  ½ **teaspoon peppermint extract**
  4 **cups skim milk**
    natural red food coloring

In a large bowl, beat together egg and honey until fluffy. Mix in peppermint extract and skim milk. Add a few drops of food coloring to obtain a light pink color.

Process mixture in an ice cream maker according to manufacturer's instructions, or turn mixture into a shallow pan and freeze until thickened but not solid. Remove from freezer, beat to break down ice crystals, and then return to freezer. Repeat this procedure twice, turning mixture into a covered container the last time. Freeze until ready to serve.

Makes 8 servings
(85 calories per serving)

Molasses Ginger Joys

Allow baking sheet to cool between batches!

  ⅓ **cup butter, softened**
  ⅓ **cup molasses**
  ⅓ **cup honey**
  1 **egg, slightly beaten**
  1¼ **cups whole wheat pastry flour**
  1¼ **cups unbleached white flour**
  1 **teaspoon baking powder**
  1 **teaspoon ground cinnamon**
  ½ **teaspoon ground ginger**

Preheat oven to 350°F. Spray a baking sheet with vegetable spray.

In a large bowl, beat together butter, molasses, and honey. Beat in egg.

In a medium-size bowl, whisk together whole wheat pastry flour, unbleached white flour, baking powder, cinnamon, and ginger. Stir into moist ingredients. Cover and chill for 1 hour.

Divide dough into fourths. Roll out 1 section between lightly floured pieces of waxed paper to an oblong about ⅛-inch thick. Cut into 2-inch circles with a cookie cutter or a juice glass. Roll out and cut second piece of dough. Place on prepared baking sheet and bake on middle shelf of oven until cookies are brown on the bottom, 5 to 8 minutes.

Cool on wire racks.

Repeat with remaining dough. Reroll scraps and make more cookies.

Makes 4 dozen cookies
(50 calories per cookie)

Apple Pear Scallop

2 apples
2 pears
⅓ cup water
2 tablespoons honey
½ teaspoon brandy extract
1 teaspoon ground cinnamon

Preheat oven to 350°F.

Peel, core, and thinly slice apples and pears. Toss with other ingredients in a 1½-quart casserole, and bake on middle shelf of oven until fruit is fork tender, about 25 minutes. Serve warm.

Makes 4 servings
(121 calories per serving)

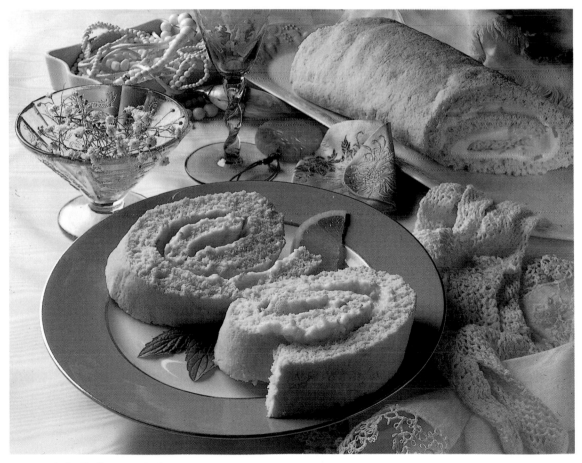

Lemon Cake Roll (page 248)

Individual Brandy Soufflés with Strawberry Sauce

3 egg whites
¼ teaspoon cream of tartar
3 tablespoons honey, divided
1 teaspoon vanilla extract
½ cup evaporated skim milk, chilled
½ teaspoon brandy extract
1 cup Strawberry Sauce (page 253)

Preheat oven to 350°F. Spray 8 8-ounce ovenproof dishes with vegetable spray.

In a medium-size bowl, beat egg whites until foamy. Add cream of tartar, 2 tablespoons of the honey, and vanilla and continue beating until stiff peaks form.

In a large bowl, beat chilled evaporated skim milk until foamy. Add remaining honey and brandy extract and continue beating until soft peaks form.

Fold beaten whites into beaten milk mixture. Turn into prepared dishes and bake on bottom shelf of oven until soufflés have risen and are lightly browned, about 15 minutes. Remove from oven. Serve immediately with 2 tablespoons of Strawberry Sauce on each soufflé.

Makes 8 servings
(77 calories per serving)

Indian Pudding

This classic dessert is traditionally baked in the oven, but I find it easier to make in an electric slow cooker.

2¼ cups skim milk
3 tablespoons honey
3 tablespoons dark molasses
⅓ cup yellow cornmeal
¼ teaspoon ground ginger
½ teaspoon ground cinnamon
¼ teaspoon ground nutmeg
⅛ teaspoon baking soda
1 egg, beaten

Lightly butter inside of electric slow cooker.

In a medium-size saucepan, scald skim milk. Stir in honey and molasses.

In a small bowl, combine cornmeal, ginger, cinnamon, nutmeg, and baking soda. Mix slowly into scalding milk, stirring constantly. Stir a little of the hot mixture into beaten egg. Return to saucepan, stirring constantly. Bring to a boil. Remove from heat and turn into prepared slow cooker. Cover and cook on low for 3 hours.

Makes 5 servings
(153 calories per serving)

Mandarin Kabobs

This is one of the few authentic Japanese desserts. But I use a honey sauce instead of the traditional Sake for dipping the orange sections.

    2 tablespoons honey, warmed
    2 tablespoons water
   24 mandarin orange sections
   ¼ cup sesame seeds
   20 mint leaves

In a small bowl, mix together honey and water. Coat orange sections with mixture then roll them in sesame seeds. Put 6 sections on each of 4 skewers, alternating with mint leaves. (Begin and end with an orange section.) Chill for several hours before serving.

Makes 4 servings
(104 calories per serving)

Strawberry Sauce

A tablespoon of this sauce dresses up plain desserts while adding only a few calories.

   1 cup unsweetened frozen
     strawberries, thawed
     and drained with juice
     reserved

   2 teaspoons cornstarch
   ¼ cup strawberry jelly

Place strawberries into a small saucepan.

Dissolve cornstarch in ¼ cup of the reserved juice. Mix into strawberries along with jelly. Bring to a boil and cook, stirring constantly, until thickened. Remove from heat, strain, and cool.

Makes about 1 cup
(10 calories per tablespoon)

Greek Yogurt Prune Pie

1 recipe for Mini Piecrust
  (page 113)
2 eggs, separated
2 tablespoons honey
1½ cups plain nonfat yogurt
1½ teaspoons vanilla extract
1½ teaspoons ground cinnamon
¼ teaspoon ground nutmeg
1 cup pitted prunes
2 tablespoons whole wheat flour
⅛ teaspoon cream of tartar

Preheat oven to 425°F.

Line a 9-inch pie plate with piecrust according to directions.

In a large bowl, beat egg yolks and honey together until light colored. Stir in yogurt, vanilla, cinnamon, and nutmeg.

In a food processor, chop prunes, adding flour to keep prune pieces separated. Stir into yogurt mixture.

In a medium-size bowl, beat egg whites until foamy. Add cream of tartar and continue beating until stiff peaks form. Fold into yogurt mixture and turn into pie shell. Bake on middle shelf of oven for 10 minutes. Reduce heat to 325°F and continue baking until filling is puffy and lightly browned, about 30 minutes. Serve warm or cold.

Makes 10 servings
(136 calories per serving)

Honey Cheese Pie

1 recipe for Mini Piecrust
  (page 113)
1 cup part-skim ricotta cheese
3 eggs
⅓ cup honey
1 cup skim milk
1½ teaspoons vanilla extract

Preheat oven to 425°F. Line a 9-inch pie plate with pastry according to directions.

In a large bowl, beat together ricotta cheese and eggs until fluffy. Beat in honey, skim milk, and vanilla. Pour into piecrust, and bake on bottom shelf of oven until a knife inserted near center comes out clean, about 30 to 35 minutes.

Makes 10 servings
(132 calories per serving)

Fluffy Grape Dessert

1 envelope unflavored gelatin
1 cup cold water
1 cup grape juice
10 seedless red grapes, quartered

In a small saucepan, sprinkle gelatin over water. Set aside for 5 minutes to soften. Heat over medium heat, stirring constantly, until gelatin dissolves. Mix in grape juice. Pour into a medium-size bowl and chill until thickened but not set, stirring occasionally so edges won't set.

Beat until about doubled in volume. Fold in grapes. Divide among 6 dessert dishes and chill until set.

Makes 6 servings
(35 calories per serving)

Creamy Carob Chip Cheesecake

32 ounces low-fat cottage cheese
⅓ cup honey
2 tablespoons unbleached white
    flour
2 tablespoons freshly squeezed
    lemon juice
2 teaspoons vanilla extract
4 eggs
½ cup carob chips, chopped

Preheat oven to 325°F. Lightly butter bottom and sides of a 9-inch springform pan.

In a food processor, blend cheese until smooth. Add remaining ingredients except carob chips through feed tube while processor is running. (If work bowl of processor is small, mix ingredients in 2 batches.) Mix in chips and pour into prepared pan. Bake on middle shelf of oven for 1 hour. Turn off heat and leave cheesecake in oven for 1 hour more. Allow to cool thoroughly.

Chill until serving time.

Makes 12 servings
(153 calories per serving)

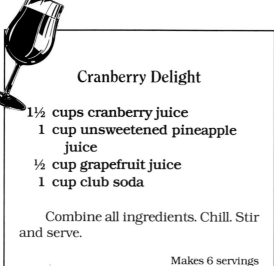

Cranberry Delight

1½ cups cranberry juice
1 cup unsweetened pineapple
    juice
½ cup grapefruit juice
1 cup club soda

Combine all ingredients. Chill. Stir and serve.

Makes 6 servings
(72 calories per serving)

Pumpkin Pineapple Pie

1 recipe for Mini Piecrust
    (page 113)
½ cup unsweetened crushed
    pineapple, well drained
1½ cups pumpkin puree
⅓ cup skim milk
3 eggs, beaten
3 tablespoons honey
1 teaspoon ground cinnamon
½ teaspoon ground ginger
½ teaspoon ground nutmeg

Bake Mini Piecrust blind according to directions.

Puree pineapple in a food processor or blender. Turn into a medium-size bowl and beat with remaining ingredients until smooth. Pour into baked pie shell. Place on middle shelf of preheated 350°F oven and bake until a knife inserted near center comes out clean, 45 to 50 minutes.

Makes 10 servings
(109 calories per serving)

Haystacks

  2 eggs
⅓ cup honey
  1 teaspoon vanilla extract
¾ cup whole wheat pastry flour
  1 cup unsweetened flaked coconut

Preheat oven to 325°F. Spray 2 baking sheets with vegetable spray.

In a medium-size bowl, beat together eggs and honey for 6 minutes. Beat in vanilla.

With a wooden spoon, gradually mix in flour. Fold in coconut and drop by teaspoonfuls about 1-inch apart on prepared baking sheets. Bake on middle shelf of oven, one batch at a time, until lightly browned, 15 to 18 minutes.

Remove to wire racks to cool.

Makes 3 dozen cookies
(29 calories per cookie)

DECEMBER

Dessert Parties—How to Show Off Your Low-Calorie Specialties

FRUIT OF THE MONTH: **GRAPES**

DESSERT OF THE MONTH: **LIGHT SPONGE CAKE**

DRINK OF THE MONTH: **EASY EGGNOG**

				1	2	3
				SMOOTH ALMOND MOUSSE	FROZEN PEPPERMINT ROLL	DEEP DISH BLUEBERRY PEAR PIE
4	**5**	**6**	**7**	**8**	**9**	**10**
EASY CHEESY DESSERT	DARLING CLEMENTINES	SPICY OATMEAL COOKIES	LIGHT SPONGE CAKE ★	FRUIT AND SHERBET PARFAITS	MARVELOUS MAPLE CREPES	FRUITED CHEESE DESSERT
11	**12**	**13**	**14**	**15**	**16**	**17**
CRAN-APPLE LOAF	PINEAPPLE GRAPE TAPIOCA	ALMOND STRAWBERRY RICE PUDDING	APRICOT RAISIN CONFECTIONS	ALMOND POTS DE CRÈME	CRANBERRY APPLESAUCE	SPECTACULAR SQUASH PIE
18	**19**	**20**	**21**	**22**	**23**	*Christmas Eve* 24
FROZEN FRUIT CUSTARD	GINGER PEARS	APPLESAUCE DROPS	BAKED BLUEBERRY WHIP	FRUITY SUNDAES	EGGNOG SOUFFLÉ	SPARKLING FRUIT TART
Christmas 25	**26**	**27**	**28**	**29**	**30**	*New Year's Eve* 31
CHRISTMAS TRIFLE	APPLE CIDER SORBET	TWENTY GRAPES	APPLE BANANA CUPCAKES	CAROB COCONUT PIE	SMOOTH STRAWBERRY PUDDING	PRETTY PARTY PUFFS

Pretty Party Puffs (page 275)

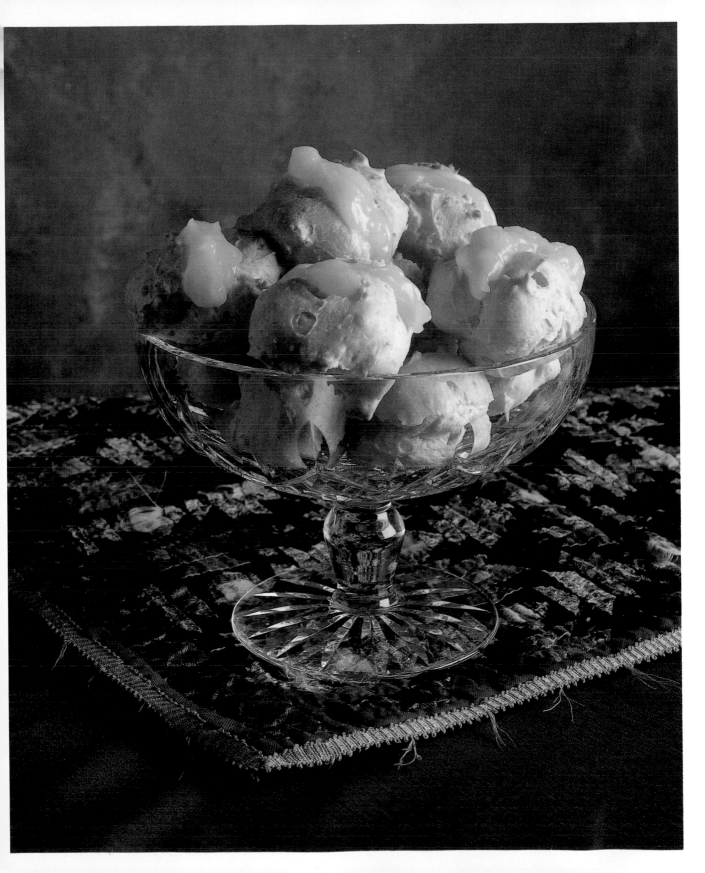

$\mathcal{D}$ecember is a festive month and a good time to discuss parties. Of course, the party suggestions in this chapter apply to other months, too.

I really enjoy a party and, if I'm to be the hostess, my favorite type is a dessert party. Just about everything can be made in advance. I bake cakes well ahead, freezing them until the day of the party, and I make pies, cookies, and confections the day before. A few hours before guests are expected, I make the punch and set the table. This leaves me free to enjoy my guests.

For this type of party, I suggest preparing a variety of desserts. Then there's no need to worry about guests' likes and dislikes. There will be something for everyone.

The success or failure of any party depends largely on the planning that goes into it. One of the cardinal rules is that your party fit the size of your home. Don't try to entertain 30 guests at a time in a tiny apartment. If there are 30 people you want to invite, have two parties, planning each group carefully.

Whether it's a sit-down affair or buffet style (the way I prefer to have dessert parties), be sure you have enough chairs for all the guests and enough small tables so that no one has to balance a plate and a glass while eating.

Plan a Perfect Setting

Although your table should look lovely, remember the desserts are the actual stars of your party. Everything else should work to show them off. A white cloth is always a safe choice, setting off both dishes and food handsomely.

Cloth napkins are much more elegant than paper ones and more substantial, too. If your party is to take place any time before dinner, choose a luncheon-size napkin of about 13 × 13 inches. But for an evening party, put out large, luxurious 22 × 22-inch napkins.

A table is more festive if it has a centerpiece. You can use one of the desserts, but I don't like to do this because as soon as the dessert is cut into, the centerpiece disappears. And some guests hesitate to help themselves to what was obviously meant to be decorative. Flowers and candles are traditional and still acceptable ornaments.

A Buffet That Works Well

A buffet party needs a planned traffic pattern that works! If the flow leads your guests to a blank wall where they must turn around, encountering other guests going in the opposite direction, you're bound to have bumps and spills. A table positioned so that guests move around it is best. Act as a guide, moving everyone in the same direction. If you do have to place the table against a wall, put candles or flowers at the back, arranging the food well toward the front where it can be easily reached.

Set your serving table so that guests come to plates, napkins, and utensils before the food. Be sure there are enough serving pieces. Every dessert should have its own.

Because your desserts will be cut into small pieces, set your table with small plates. You don't want a piece of cake to look lost on a huge plate. I use small, four-ounce beverage glasses too. Guests return for further helpings if they desire.

Don't crowd your table with more desserts and drinks than it can accommodate without looking crowded. Not only is it unattractive, it is difficult for guests to help themselves to the food. Set up another table if necessary. I usually have the beverage in a separate place.

Serve a wide variety of different, yet compatible desserts. For instance, if you're serving two cakes and one's a carob tube cake, make the other one a lemon cake roll, or a pumpkin cake. And a chiffon pie would go well with a pastry of a different texture, like fruit. For a party of this type, I select desserts without gooey fillings or runny sauces. To top it off, I include a punch that won't overpower the dessert flavors. I always serve punch at parties. This eliminates the need to find out the beverage preference of each guest and then prepare it. (You'll find several of my favorite punch recipes throughout the book.) And, of course, I make sure to have a large supply of ice on hand.

If one of the desserts you're serving is chilled, place it over a bowl of ice to keep it fresh. But be sure it's securely set and not precariously balanced on the ice. Set out pads for hot desserts.

I always plan at least three pieces of dessert for each person. It isn't my job as hostess to police the calorie intake of my guests. I provide low calorie desserts; how much they eat is up to them. And, yes, I usually do have leftovers, but I wrap them up and tuck them into the freezer for future use.

I slice all the desserts for a buffet into small pieces before I put them on the table. And I put the first piece (the most difficult to remove) on a plate beside the rest of the dessert.

An open house presents food problems. If guests will be dropping in at different times, don't put all the desserts out at once. Save a surprise or two for the middle of the party. You don't want your desserts to look wilted or picked over when the last of your guests arrive.

With delicious diet desserts, a carefully planned table setting, and congenial guests, your party is bound to be a success.

Smooth Almond Mousse

2 cups part-skim ricotta cheese
¼ cup skim milk
2 tablespoons honey
2 teaspoons vanilla extract
1½ teaspoons almond extract
½ teaspoon ground cinnamon

In a food processor, combine all ingredients. Divide among 4 dessert dishes and chill for several hours before serving.

Makes 4 servings
(129 calories per serving)

Frozen Peppermint Roll

1 recipe for Jelly Roll Cake
    (page 54)
1 recipe for French Peppermint Ice
    Milk (page 250), softened
¼ cup Coconut Sugar (page 66)

Bake Jelly Roll Cake according to directions.

Quickly spread softened ice milk over cake. Sprinkle with Coconut Sugar. Roll up from narrow end and place, seam side down, on plastic wrap. Wrap roll. Wrap again in foil and freeze.

Take out of freezer 10 minutes before serving and remove outer wrap.

Makes 12 servings
(151 calories per serving)

Deep Dish Blueberry Pear Pie

This pie will be easier to slice cold than hot.

6 fresh pears
8 cups water
1 tablespoon freshly squeezed
    lemon juice
2 cups unsweetened frozen blue-
    berries, thawed
¼ cup honey
1 tablespoon cornstarch
1 teaspoon ground ginger
1 recipe for Skinny Piecrust
    (page 6)

Preheat oven to 400°F. Spray bottom of a 10-inch pie plate with vegetable spray.

Peel, core, and thinly slice pears, dropping them into water mixed with lemon juice to prevent discoloration.

Drain pear slices. In a large bowl, toss them with remaining ingredients except piecrust. Turn into prepared pie plate.

Roll out piecrust and place it over filling, crimping edges over rim of pie plate. Cut vents in piecrust and bake on middle shelf of oven for 50 minutes. If crust is browning too fast, cover it with foil and continue baking.

Makes 10 servings
(149 calories per serving)

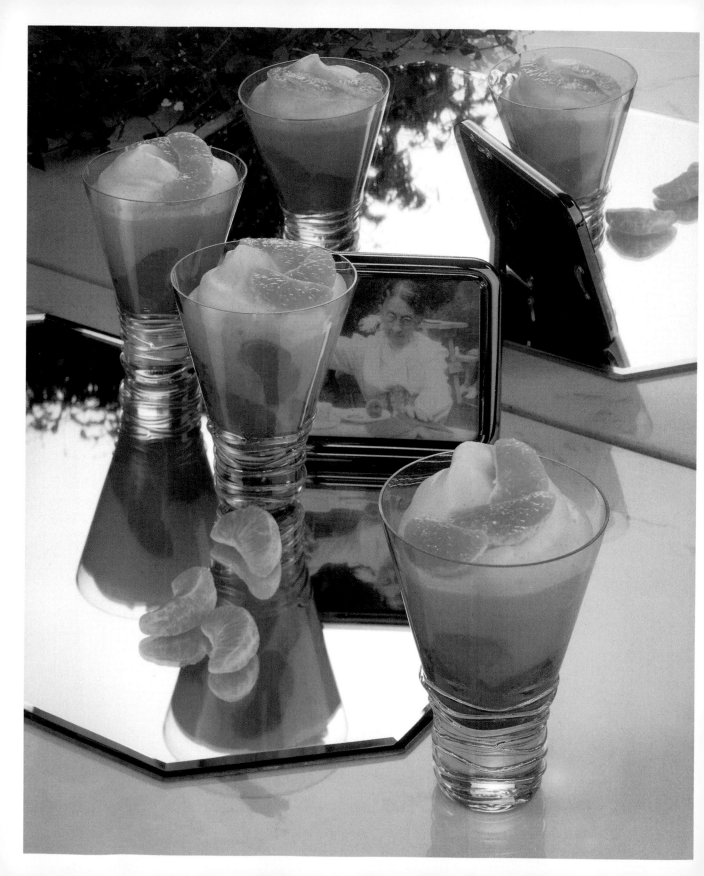

Darling Clementines

If the clementines are difficult to find,
you may use seedless oranges instead.

1 envelope unflavored gelatin
1 cup water, divided
3 tablespoons honey, divided
1 cup freshly squeezed orange juice
1 teaspoon orange extract
½ cup evaporated skim milk, chilled
½ teaspoon ground cinnamon
1 teaspoon vanilla extract
3 clementines

In a small saucepan, sprinkle gelatin over ½ cup of the water. Set aside to soften for 5 minutes. Heat, stirring constantly, until gelatin dissolves. Stir in 2 tablespoons of the honey, remaining water, orange juice, and orange extract. Chill until very thick but not set.

In a medium-size bowl, beat evaporated skim milk until foamy. Add cinnamon, vanilla, and remaining honey. Continue beating until soft peaks form. Beat in gelatin mixture.

Peel clementines and separate into sections. Cut sections into halves and divide among 6 dessert glasses. Top each with gelatin mixture and chill until set.

Makes 6 servings
(105 calories per serving)

Spicy Oatmeal Cookies

¼ cup butter, softened
⅓ cup honey
1 egg
1 teaspoon vanilla extract
½ cup whole wheat pastry flour
½ cup unbleached white flour
⅔ cup rolled oats
¼ teaspoon baking powder
¼ teaspoon baking soda
2 teaspoons ground cinnamon
½ teaspoon ground nutmeg
¼ cup raisins, plumped

Preheat oven to 350°F.

In a medium-size bowl, beat butter until fluffy. Beat in honey, then egg and vanilla.

In a medium-size bowl, whisk together dry ingredients. Stir in raisins and mix into moist ingredients.

Drop by rounded teaspoonfuls onto 2 ungreased baking sheets. Bake each batch on middle shelf of oven until golden, 8 to 10 minutes.

Makes 30 cookies
(57 calories per cookie)

Darling Clementines (on this page)

★ Light Sponge Cake

*This versatile cake lends itself to any
number of toppings.*

½ cup whole wheat pastry flour
½ cup unbleached white flour
6 eggs, separated
¼ teaspoon cream of tartar
1½ tablespoons water
⅔ cup honey
2 teaspoons vanilla extract
1 cup Mock Whipped Cream
(page 10), divided
12 seedless green or red grapes

Preheat oven to 350°F. Line bottom
of an 11½ × 7½-inch pan with parchment paper.

Sift together whole wheat pastry flour
and unbleached white flour.

In a large bowl, beat egg whites until
foamy. Add cream of tartar and continue
beating until stiff peaks form.

In a small bowl, beat egg yolks and
water until lemon colored. Drizzle in
honey and beat until mixture doubles
in volume. Mix in vanilla. Fold flour into
egg yolks. Fold batter into egg whites.
Spoon into prepared pan and bake until
cake springs back when lightly pressed,
20 to 25 minutes.

Invert, placing edges of cake pan on
2 glass bowls. When cool remove from
pan and carefully strip off paper.

Just before serving, put a dollop of
Mock Whipped Cream and a grape on
each piece of cake.

*Makes 12 servings
(146 calories per serving)*

Fruited Cheese Dessert

1⅓ cups part-skim ricotta cheese
¼ cup honey
1 teaspoon vanilla extract
1 cup sliced unsweetened frozen
strawberries
½ cup quartered seedless green
grapes
4 teaspoons ground pecans

Thoroughly blend together ricotta
cheese, honey, and vanilla. Fold in strawberries and grapes. Divide among 4 dessert dishes. Sprinkle pecans on top.

*Makes 4 servings
(98 calories per serving)*

Cran-Apple Loaf

1 Lazy Day Loaf Cake (page 201)
1 cup Cranberry Applesauce
(page 268)
¼ cup Coconut Sugar (page 66)

Split cake in half, lengthwise. Spread
sauce on lower half and put upper half
on top of sauce. Sprinkle with Coconut
Sugar.

*Makes 12 servings
(114 calories per serving)*

Fruit and Sherbet Parfaits

This lovely blending of flavors makes an elegant company dessert.

1 pint Raspberry Rum Sherbet
  (page 165)
1 ripe honeydew melon
1 pint fresh blueberries
  mint leaves, optional

With a melon baller, make small balls of Raspberry Rum Sherbet, placing them on a baking sheet lined with waxed paper. Cover with waxed paper and place in freezer.

Halve melon and scoop out seeds. Make melon balls with melon baller. Chill.

Just before serving, divide ingredients among 8 parfait glasses, alternating melon and blueberries with sherbet in several layers. Decorate with mint leaves, if desired. Serve immediately.

Makes 8 servings
(179 calories per serving)

Marvelous Maple Crepes

¾ cup part-skim ricotta cheese
1 cup low-fat cottage cheese
1 tablespoon honey
3 tablespoons maple syrup, divided
1½ teaspoons vanilla extract
8 Delicious Diet Crepes (page 33)
½ cup plain low-fat yogurt
  ground cinnamon for sprinkling

In a medium-size bowl, beat together ricotta cheese, cottage cheese, honey, 1 tablespoon of the maple syrup, and vanilla. If mixture is runny, chill it until it thickens.

Divide mixture among crepes, spreading it on tops, and fold each in half.

In a small bowl, stir remaining maple syrup into yogurt. Spoon over crepes, sprinkle with cinnamon, and serve immediately.

Makes 8 servings
(126 calories per serving)

Cranberry Applesauce

1 tablespoon cornstarch
¾ cup water
¾ cup fresh cranberries
2 tablespoons honey
1 teaspoon freshly squeezed lemon
    juice
1 teaspoon ground cinnamon
2 apples
1 teaspoon vanilla extract

Dissolve cornstarch in water. Pour into medium-size saucepan. Add cranberries, honey, lemon juice, and cinnamon.

Peel, core, and chop apples, stirring them into cranberry mixture as you chop them. Bring to a boil, stirring constantly. Reduce heat and simmer, stirring often, until cranberries burst and mixture thickens, about 15 minutes. Stir in vanilla.

Makes 2 cups
(64 calories per cup)

Pineapple Grape Tapioca

¾ cup unsweetened pineapple juice
2 teaspoons honey
¼ cup quick-cooking tapioca
1 teaspoon vanilla extract
1 egg yolk
1¼ cups skim milk
2 egg whites
⅛ teaspoon cream of tartar
20 seedless green grapes,
    quartered

Pour pineapple juice into a medium-size saucepan. Mix in honey. Sprinkle tapioca over top and set aside to soften for 5 minutes. Bring to a boil over medium heat stirring constantly. Stir in vanilla. Remove from heat.

In a small bowl, beat egg yolk and skim milk together. Put a little of the hot mixture into beaten yolk. Return to pan, whisking to blend. Cook over low heat, whisking constantly, until mixture thickens, about 10 minutes. Remove from heat and let cool.

In a medium-size bowl, beat egg whites until foamy. Add cream of tartar and continue beating until stiff peaks form. Fold into cooled tapioca. Chill.

When ready to serve, fold in grapes.

Makes 8 servings
(62 calories per serving)

Apricot Raisin Confections

1 cup unsweetened flaked coconut,
    divided
1 cup dried apricots
¼ cup raisins
1 tablespoon honey
2 teaspoons freshly squeezed
    orange juice

In a food processor, process ½ cup of the coconut until it is coconut sugar. Set aside on a plate.

Process remaining ingredients in food processor. Roll mixture into balls of about 1 tablespoon each between palms of hands. Roll balls in coconut sugar.

Makes 32 cookies
(25 calories per cookie)

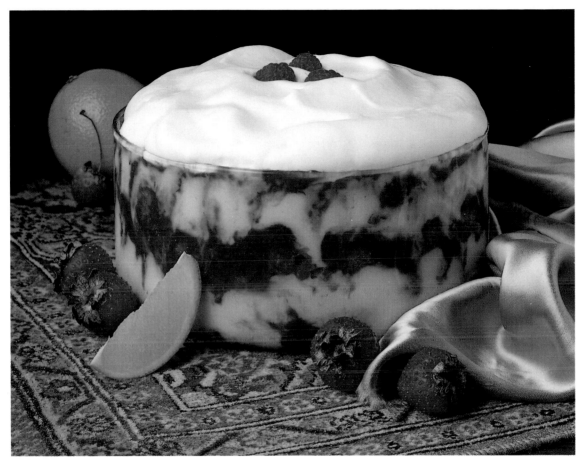

Christmas Trifle (page 274)

Easy Cheesy Dessert

2 cups low-fat cottage cheese
¼ cup honey
¼ teaspoon ground cinnamon
1 teaspoon vanilla extract
½ cup Perfect Pineapple Sauce
   (page 60), divided

In a food processor or an electric mixer, beat together cottage cheese, honey, cinnamon, and vanilla until smooth. Divide among 4 sherbet glasses. Cover with plastic wrap and chill well.

Serve each portion topped with 2 tablespoons of the sauce.

Makes 4 servings
(175 calories per serving)

Slim Pastry Cream

½ envelope unflavored gelatin
½ cup cold water
1 cup skim milk, divided
1 tablespoon cornstarch

2 egg yolks
3 tablespoons honey
1 teaspoon vanilla extract

In a small saucepan, sprinkle gelatin over cold water. Set aside to soften for 5 minutes.

In a medium-size saucepan, heat ¾ cup of the skim milk. Shake remaining skim milk and cornstarch together in a jar with a tight-fitting lid, or whisk together until well blended.

In a small bowl, beat egg yolks and honey together until lemon colored. Beat in cornstarch mixture.

Pour hot skim milk into the top of a double boiler and set over hot water. Slowly whisk in egg yolk mixture and cook, stirring constantly, until custard coats the back of a wooden spoon. Remove from heat and pour into a medium-size bowl.

Heat softened gelatin until dissolved. Stir into pastry cream. Mix in vanilla. Allow to cool before using.

Makes about 1½ cups
(19 calories per tablespoon)

Almond Pots de Crème

½ cup instant nonfat dry milk
2 cups boiling water
2 tablespoons honey
1 teaspoon almond extract
1 teaspoon vanilla extract
3 eggs, beaten

Preheat oven to 350°F.
In a medium-size bowl, dissolve nonfat dry milk in water. Add honey and extracts, stirring to blend. Pour a little of the mixture into beaten eggs, whisking well. Return to bowl, whisking constantly. Pour into 6 ovenproof cups and put in shallow pan on middle shelf of oven. Pour water into pan until it reaches halfway up the sides of cups. Bake until just set, about 30 minutes.
Chill before serving.

Makes 6 servings
(94 calories per serving)

Spectacular Squash Pie

1 recipe for Skinny Piecrust
   (page 6)
2 eggs
1 10-ounce package frozen squash,
   thawed
⅓ cup honey
½ teaspoon vanilla extract
1 cup skim milk, divided
2 tablespoons cornstarch
2 teaspoons ground cinnamon
¾ teaspoon ground nutmeg

Preheat oven to 350°F. Line a 9-inch pie plate with pastry and set aside.
In a large bowl, beat eggs. Add squash, honey, and vanilla and beat to mix well.
In a jar with a tight-fitting lid, shake together ½ cup of the skim milk, cornstarch, and spices. Mix into squash. Stir in remaining milk. Turn into piecrust and bake on bottom shelf of oven until filling is set and crust is browned, 55 to 60 minutes.
Cool before serving.

Makes 10 servings
(118 calories per serving)

Almond Strawberry Rice Pudding

1¼ cups skim milk
2 tablespoons honey
2 eggs, beaten
1 teaspoon vanilla extract
¼ teaspoon almond extract
2 cups cooked rice
1 cup fresh or unsweetened frozen strawberries, quartered

Preheat oven to 325°F. Spray a 1½-quart casserole with vegetable spray.
In a large bowl, beat together skim milk, honey, eggs, and extracts. Stir in rice and fold in berries. Bake on middle shelf of oven until set near, but not in, the center, about 45 minutes.
Allow to cool before serving.

Makes 8 servings
(95 calories per serving)

Applesauce Drops

¼ cup butter, softened
¼ cup cream cheese, softened
⅓ cup honey
1 egg
1½ teaspoons vanilla extract
1 cup whole wheat pastry flour
1 cup unbleached white flour
1 teaspoon baking powder
1 tablespoon ground cinnamon
½ teaspoon ground nutmeg
1½ cups Applesauce (page 90)
1 cup rolled oats

Preheat oven to 350°F. Spray a baking sheet with vegetable spray.

In a large bowl, beat together butter, cream cheese, and honey. Beat in egg and vanilla.

Into a medium-size bowl, sift together whole wheat pastry flour, unbleached white flour, baking powder, cinnamon, and nutmeg. Whisk to blend.

In another medium-size bowl, mix together Applesauce and rolled oats. Mix into moist ingredients. Stir in flour mixture and drop batter by heaping teaspoonfuls onto prepared baking sheet. Bake, one batch at a time, on middle shelf of oven until browned on the bottoms, 15 to 18 minutes.

Cool on wire racks. Bake second batch on cooled baking sheet.

Makes 5 dozen cookies
(37 calories per cookie)

Frozen Fruit Custard

2 cups evaporated skim milk, chilled
2 tablespoons honey
1 teaspoon vanilla extract
1½ teaspoons rum extract
2 cups Slim Pastry Cream (page 270)
¼ cup chopped dates
¼ cup raisins, plumped
¼ cup unsweetened flaked coconut

Lightly oil a 12-cup ring mold or bundt pan.

In a large bowl, beat evaporated skim milk until soft peaks form. Continue beating, drizzling in honey and extracts. Fold in pastry cream, dates, raisins, and coconut. Turn into prepared mold or pan, cover, and freeze.

To unmold, dip bottom of mold in warm water for 60 seconds. Unmold on a plate and slice with a warm, sharp knife.

Makes 10 servings
(142 calories per serving)

Fruity Sundaes

1 large banana
1 cup unsweetened frozen melon
   balls, thawed
8 seedless green or red grapes,
   halved
1½ cups unsweetened frozen raspberries, thawed, divided
2 cups Vanilla Ice Milk (page 79),
   divided

Slice banana into a medium-size bowl. Mix in melon balls, grapes, and 1 cup of the raspberries. Divide mixture among 4 dessert dishes. Top each with ½ cup of the Vanilla Ice Milk. Divide remaining raspberries among dishes, spooning them over ice milk. Serve immediately.

*Makes 4 servings
(192 calories per serving)*

Baked Blueberry Whip

This dish is reminiscent of a soufflé in texture, but this meringue-based dessert doesn't rise as high or collapse as low as a classic soufflé.

1½ cups fresh or unsweetened frozen blueberries, thawed
½ cup grape juice
1½ tablespoons cornstarch
½ cup water
2 tablespoons honey, divided
4 egg whites
¼ teaspoon cream of tartar

In a medium-size saucepan, combine blueberries and grape juice. Dissolve cornstarch in water and mix into blueberry mixture. Stir in 1 tablespoon of the honey and cook over medium heat, stirring constantly, until mixture bubbles and thickens. Remove from heat and set aside to cool.

Preheat oven to 325°F. Spray a 2-quart casserole with vegetable spray.

In a large bowl, beat egg whites until foamy. Add cream of tartar and remaining honey and continue beating until stiff peaks form. Fold into cooled blueberry mixture. Turn into prepared casserole and bake on middle shelf of oven for 30 minutes. Serve warm.

*Makes 10 servings
(46 calories per serving)*

Eggnog Soufflé

1 envelope unflavored gelatin
1 cup skim milk
¼ cup honey
4 eggs, separated
1 teaspoon vanilla extract
½ teaspoon rum extract
¼ teaspoon cream of tartar
½ teaspoon ground nutmeg

Lightly oil a 4-cup soufflé dish and fit it with a soufflé collar.*

In a medium-size saucepan, sprinkle gelatin over skim milk. Set aside to soften for 5 minutes. Add honey and heat over medium heat just until gelatin dissolves.

In a small bowl, beat egg yolks. Add a little of the hot milk mixture, stirring constantly. Gradually return to hot milk and cook, stirring constantly, until mixture thickens enough to coat the back of a metal spoon. Remove from heat. Stir in vanilla and rum extracts and chill until thickened but not set.

In a medium-size bowl, beat egg whites until foamy. Add cream of tartar and continue beating until stiff peaks form. Fold into gelatin mixture and turn into soufflé dish. Chill until set.

Before serving, remove soufflé collar and sprinkle top of soufflé with nutmeg.

Makes 8 servings
(87 calories per serving)

*To make a soufflé collar, cut a piece of foil 10 inches wide and long enough to encircle soufflé dish plus 2 inches. Fold lengthwise. Tie collar around dish with string, allowing foil to extend 3 inches above rim. Tape seam together. Butter or oil inside of collar.

Christmas Trifle

This is a happy ending for a Christmas gathering.

20 Ladyfingers (page 108)
½ cup Strawberry Sauce (page 253)
3 cups Very Vanilla Pudding (page 84), divided
¾ cup seedless green grapes, halved
½ cup unsweetened frozen raspberries, thawed
¾ cup mandarin orange sections, halved
½ cup evaporated skim milk, chilled
1 tablespoon honey

Line bottom of a 2-quart glass bowl with half of the Ladyfingers. Drizzle Strawberry Sauce over them. Make a layer of 1½ cups vanilla pudding.

In a medium-size bowl, toss fruit together. Arrange half of it on top of the pudding. Repeat layers. Refrigerate for at least 2 hours.

At serving time, beat evaporated skim milk in a small bowl until foamy. Add honey and beat until soft peaks form. Spread on top of trifle and serve immediately.

Makes 12 servings
(174 calories per serving)

Sparkling Fruit Tart

1 recipe for **Skinny Piecrust**
   (page 6)
1 cup creamed cottage cheese
1 cup **Slim Pastry Cream**
   (page 270)
½ teaspoon almond extract
1 medium-size banana
2 kiwi fruits
2 fresh peaches
1 tablespoon freshly squeezed
   lemon juice
¼ cup red currant jelly

Bake piecrust according to directions. Cool.

In a medium-size bowl, beat together cottage cheese, pastry cream, and almond extract. Spread on bottom of prepared piecrust.

Peel and thinly slice all fruit. Halve kiwi slices. Arrange fruit decoratively on top of cheese mixture. Brush bananas and peaches lightly with lemon juice to prevent discoloration.

In a small saucepan, melt currant jelly. Brush on all fruit. Serve immediately.

Makes 12 servings
(129 calories per serving)

Pretty Party Puffs

A crowd-pleasing dessert!

¾ cup whole wheat pastry flour
¾ cup unbleached white flour
1¼ cups water
¼ cup butter
4 eggs, slightly beaten
2 cups Sunshine Filling (page 180),
   divided

Preheat oven to 400°F.

In a medium-size bowl, sift together whole wheat pastry flour and unbleached white flour, whisking to blend.

Put water and butter into a medium-size saucepan and bring to a rolling boil. Reduce heat and stir in flour, beating with a wooden spoon until mixture pulls away from sides of pan. Remove from heat and set aside to cool slightly.

Add eggs, 1 at a time, beating until smooth. Drop batter by slightly mounded teaspoonfuls onto an ungreased baking sheet. Bake on middle shelf of oven for about 20 minutes, or until lightly browned.

Pierce sides of each puff with tip of a sharp knife to release steam and place puffs on wire racks to cool.

When cool, split each puff crosswise with a sharp knife, removing any soft or uncooked dough. Fill each puff with 2 teaspoons of filling and replace tops. To serve, pile in a pyramid on a large plate.

Makes about 4 dozen puffs
(40 calories per puff)

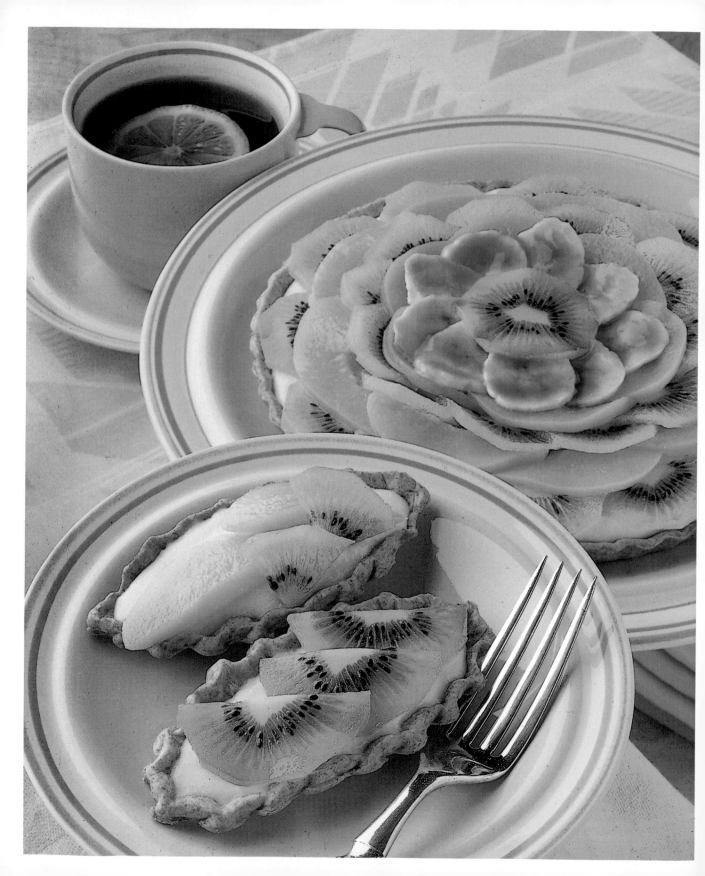

Carob Coconut Pie

2¼ cups skim milk, divided
1½ envelopes unflavored gelatin,
      divided
  1 cup part-skim ricotta cheese
  ¼ cup plus 1 tablespoon honey,
      divided
  2 teaspoons vanilla extract, divided
  ¼ cup carob chips
  2 tablespoons butter
  1 tablespoon cornstarch
  ½ cup unsweetened flaked coconut

Spray a 9-inch deep-dish pie plate with vegetable spray.

In a small saucepan, sprinkle ½ envelope of the gelatin over ¼ cup of the skim milk. Set aside to soften for 5 minutes.

In a medium-size bowl, beat together ricotta, ¼ cup of the honey, and 1 teaspoon of the vanilla until smooth.

In the top of a double boiler set over hot water, melt together carob chips and butter.

Heat softened gelatin mixture over medium heat stirring constantly, until gelatin dissolves. Beat gelatin mixture, along with carob mixture, into cheese mixture and spread on bottom of prepared pie plate. Chill until set.

In a medium-size saucepan, dissolve cornstarch in 1 cup of the skim milk. Sprinkle remaining gelatin over top and set aside to soften for 5 minutes. Add remaining honey and cook over medium heat, stirring constantly, until mixture thickens slightly and gelatin dissolves. Stir in remaining vanilla, remaining skim milk, and coconut. Gently pour over top of carob mixture and chill until set.

Makes 10 servings
(166 calories per serving)

Apple Cider Sorbet

  3 cups apple cider
1½ teaspoons ground cinnamon
  2 tablespoons honey
  1 cup hot water

Pour cider into a large bowl. Dissolve cinnamon and honey in hot water. Add to cider.

Process mixture in an ice cream maker according to manufacturer's instructions, or turn mixture into a large shallow pan and freeze until mushy. Remove from freezer, beat to break down ice crystals, and then return to freezer. Repeat this procedure twice, putting sorbet in a covered container the last time. Freeze until ready to serve.

Makes 8 servings
(60 calories per serving)

Sparkling Fruit Tart (page 275)

Apple Banana Cupcakes

1 6-ounce can unsweetened frozen
　　apple juice concentrate, thawed
2 ripe bananas, chunked
2 eggs
2 tablespoons honey
1 teaspoon vanilla extract
1 cup whole wheat pastry flour
1 cup unbleached white flour
2 teaspoons baking powder
1 teaspoon ground cinnamon

Preheat oven to 350°F. Line a 12-cup muffin tin with paper liners.

In a food processor, blend apple juice, bananas, eggs, honey, and vanilla until smooth.

Into a medium-size bowl, sift together remaining ingredients. Stir with a wire whisk to blend well.

In a large bowl, stir together both mixtures until well blended. Turn into prepared muffin cups, filling to tops, and bake on middle shelf of oven for 20 minutes.

Makes 12 servings
(146 calories per serving)

Smooth Strawberry Pudding

2 envelopes unflavored gelatin
½ cup cold water
1 cup skim milk
3 tablespoons honey
1½ teaspoons vanilla extract
4 cups unsweetened frozen straw-
　　berries, thawed
8 mint leaves, optional

In a medium-size saucepan, sprinkle gelatin over water. Set aside for 5 minutes to soften. Add skim milk and honey and heat over medium heat, stirring constantly, until gelatin dissolves. Remove from heat and stir in vanilla.

In a food processor, puree strawberries. Add gelatin mixture and process until just blended. Divide among 8 dessert glasses and chill until set.

Decorate with mint leaves before serving, if desired.

Makes 8 servings
(68 calories per serving)

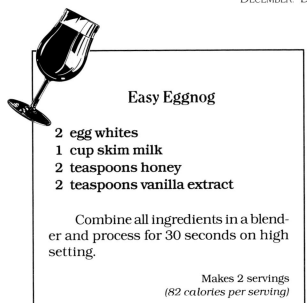

Easy Eggnog

2 egg whites
1 cup skim milk
2 teaspoons honey
2 teaspoons vanilla extract

Combine all ingredients in a blender and process for 30 seconds on high setting.

Makes 2 servings
(82 calories per serving)

Ginger Pears

6 firm ripe pears
¼ cup honey
⅓ cup hot water
¼ teaspoon ground ginger
1 tablespoon butter

Preheat oven to 350°F.

Peel, halve, and core pears. Arrange in a large casserole.

In a small bowl, mix together honey, hot water, and ginger. Pour over pears and dot with butter. Cover and bake on middle shelf of oven for 30 minutes.

Makes 6 servings
(160 calories per serving)

Index

Page references in **boldface** type refer to photographs.